The Witch
in the
Waiting Room

The Witch

in the
Waiting Room

A PHYSICIAN EXAMINES
PARANORMAL PHENOMENA
IN MEDICINE

Robert S. Bobrow, M.D.

THUNDER'S MOUTH PRESS • NEW YORK

THE WITCH IN THE WAITING ROOM:
A Physician Examines Paranormal Phenomena In Medicine

Published by
Thunder's Mouth Press
An Imprint of Avalon Publishing Group Inc.
245 West 17th Street, 11th Floor
New York, NY 10011

AVALON
publishing group incorporated

Library of Congress Cataloging-in-Publication Data is available.

ISBN-10: 1-56025-814-4
ISBN-13: 978-1-56025-814-8

9 8 7 6 5 4 3 2 1

Book design by Bettina Wilhelm
Printed in the United States of America
Distributed by Publishers Group West

For Ellen, Jennifer, and Heather,
who were with me all the way

Contents

Part 2

Acknowledgments

This book would never have come to exist were it not for the following people who took it seriously, in order:

Douglas Gasner, the late Jack Froom and the family medicine department at Stony Brook University, Claudia Dowling, John Moffett, Dorothy Leeds, Sharyn Kolberg, my agent Gary Heidt, and Jofie Ferrari-Adler, who originally accepted the proposal.

I would like to thank the following people for taking the time to speak to me: Marsha Adams, Robert O. Becker, Larry Dossey, Bruce Greyson, Vernon M. Neppe, Michael A. Persinger, and David Shalloway.

And for answering e-mails, sharing stories, or otherwise contributing: Carlos S. Alvarado, Mitch Bobrow, Stephen Engel,

Valerie Feldman, Joan Fusco, Yuri Gorokhova, Diane Interbartolo, Danielle Long, Rich Murdocco, Naomi Norman, Karl Pribram, Dean Radin, Nancy Raphael, Glen Rein, Oleg Reznik, R. Mark Sadler, Manal Soliman, and Dennis Totino.

How This Book Came to be Written

The paranormal is what lies beyond the reach of current scientific explanation. Telepathy, reincarnation, UFO phenomena, and witchcraft are a few examples. I myself have never experienced anything paranormal. My interest derives from a general curiosity of all things medical. I became a generalist physician so I wouldn't have to exclude anything from my field of study. Along the years of medical practice I collected, as many of my colleagues do, articles of interest from the medical literature: things that would be relevant to patients' illnesses, or other medical-science items I thought worth noting. My antennae must have been tuned to the slightly unusual, as my collection included data that claimed that water pills prevented osteoporosis and that cigarette smoking reduced the incidence of ulcerative colitis or Parkinson's disease, and data about how donating blood prevented heart attacks. But also, among the many papers I had clipped out, there was research including: a case of a serious disease called lupus being cured by witchcraft; a woman with voices in her head telling her she had a brain tumor, who had exactly that; and a man so convinced he was a cat that no psychiatrist's therapy could change this belief.

As a member of an academic department in a medical school (Department of Family Medicine, Stony Brook University), I was required to give a Grand Rounds presentation about once a year. This was a one-and-a-half-hour lecture to medical students, departmental faculty, and anyone else interested, given each week as part of a medical school's general didactics. I was usually allowed to choose my own topic; and one year, when the time came, I asked if I could talk about paranormal phenomena depicted in the medical literature, and got an okay. There were enough articles already within my collection to form a lecture base. In reality, I just thought it would be more fun to prepare and deliver a lecture on paranormality, rather than on a stolid, "normal" subject like asthma or heart failure.

The lectures begin at 8 A.M. on a Wednesday, to a barely awake audience, many of whom are only there because they have to be there. I had some trepidation about presenting what is often considered as anti-science to this conventional medical-school gathering. But my talk was quite well received, and I was surprised by what happened afterward: Several members of the department approached me, including the chairman, and told me about paranormal experiences they or a member of their families had had. Buoyed by this unexpected interest in the subject, I wrote up the lecture as a medical paper, and it was published by the British journal *Medical Hypotheses;* that paper is now expanded into this book.

Perhaps I should not have been surprised by the audience reaction, medical sophisticates that they were. The number of Americans holding at least one paranormal belief has increased sharply during the last twenty-five years, for reasons unknown, to a level where a majority of our population now accepts at least one such belief. In a *Newsweek*-sponsored 1996 poll, two thirds of respondents believed the power of extra-sensory perception (ESP) to be real; a Gallup poll the same year found that 72 percent of Americans believed in the literal existence of angels.[1] In Great Britain, the situation is similar: In a 1997 survey, seven out of ten people believed in some form of paranormal activity. And in 1998, a majority of responders believed in telepathy and ESP.[2] A 2005 Gallup survey[3] finds that about three-quarters of Americans hold some paranormal belief. One has only to look at the TV listings on any evening to see that Americans have a hearty appetite for the paranormal.

My chairman used the occasion of my lecture to tell me about his seven-year-old son, who "saw" his missing cat in a basement room with an old man and other cats. This turned out to be correct—an elderly man on the block took in strays, and their lost cat was mistaken for one. The little boy had also "known" that his friend in Paris was suddenly in distress. This was also correct—the friend, at the time, was being rushed to the hospital with appendicitis.

One of the senior resident physicians, who had a Ph.D. in microbiology—i.e., a research scientist—approached me after the lecture to say that while she generally had no patience with

1 Goode, E. *Paranormal Beliefs*, pp. 2, 117. Prospect Heights: Waveland Press, 2000.

2 *Market & Opinion Research International*, MORI House, London.

3 gallup.com (accessed 11/17/05).

"this sort of thing," she did find my presentation interesting and well researched. Four months later, at the residents' graduation party, I happened to be sitting at a table with her and her family. It came out that I had lectured on paranormal phenomena, and her sister remarked: "Did you tell him about Uncle Jack?" Their uncle, it seemed, had some sort of precognitive power that was noted when they all drove in a car together, the uncle calling out the descriptions of automobiles that had not yet appeared, but would do so shortly.

Another time, I was working at a public health clinic, when one of the nurses noticed a book on my desk about some paranormal subject. She asked what my opinion was, and I said I was researching it open-mindedly. She came closer, looked behind her to make sure no one else was listening, and proceeded to tell me about two unusual experiences: the time her father saw a UFO while driving home from work one night, and the time she knew exactly when a cancer patient with whom she had been very involved had died. These were things she rarely shared.

I wonder how many other colleagues, given the opportunity, would validate those poll results.

What Is In the Book?

The United States' National Library of Medicine, based in Bethesda, Maryland, holds the world's largest medical library. Its database contains references, and often abstracts, for over 4,600 scholarly biomedical journals covering medicine and related fields, the journals having been chosen by a chartered advisory committee. Not all published journals are included; the *Paranormal Research Journal* and *The Journal of the Society of Psychical Research,* for example, are not. The implication is that the journals that *are* included meet certain standards for objective review and accuracy.

The National Library's database is loosely known as "the medical literature." It is our profession's Gospel, from which all our knowledge derives, from which our textbooks are largely written. Originally known as the Medical Literature Analysis and Retrieval System (MEDLARS), it went on-line when computers made this possible; MEDLARS on-line is called MEDLINE.

MEDLINE is accessible by computer for free at pubmed.gov. The bulk of the database dates back to 1966, but citations sometimes go back to the 1950s. The citations and, frequently, the article abstracts can be retrieved using author, journal title, article title, or subject matter in the search. Most of the research described in this book comes from MEDLINE; that which does not is taken from published works of physicians where I believed the reportage to be meticulous and accurate. All journals referenced in this book are in MEDLINE, unless otherwise stated. Since MEDLINE does not contain a subject matter heading (search term) for "paranormal phenomena," articles were retrieved using individual search words such as "psychic," "witchcraft," or "parapsychology." A number of relevant pieces, although indexed in MEDLINE, would not have been found via search words.

So this book is primarily a compendium of physician-described patient phenomena, where both patient and physician are a bit bewildered about what has happened. Paranormal items not discussed—e.g., communication with the dead—are omitted because I could not find what I considered to be scholarly research on these subjects. The book is not intended to be comprehensive, as there is no all-inclusive medical database to search. These are only interesting pieces of a puzzle that will someday be put together.

Where research into the seemingly paranormal turns up a logical explanation, this will also be presented. Observed phenomena are explained when they can be, or described as accurately as possible when they cannot be, in the hope that in the future, as science advances, understanding will follow.

Remember that what is paranormal in one era may become mainstream science in another: A radio in Abraham Lincoln's time would have been perceived as a talking box—nothing more, nothing less, and totally incomprehensible. Acupuncture, endorsed by the government's National Institutes of Health (NIH) at a 1998 consensus conference, at least for efficacy in some pain syndromes, was considered beyond believability and reason when the first reports of pins in the skin providing surgical anesthesia trickled West only forty years ago. Observations that don't make scientific sense today need not be swept under a carpet of denial; tomorrow is another day.

Part I

One

Perspective I: The World We Live In

We all know that the earth is round. We grew up knowing it. Yet the surface of the earth appears flat and for centuries many believed this to be reality. Astute observations, however, suggested otherwise: Ships sailing away disappeared from the bottom up, and sooner to an observer at sea level than to one atop a mountain; the sun cast shadows of different lengths at different latitudes on the same day at the same time; the earth's shadow upon the moon during a lunar eclipse was curved.

What is weird about a spherical earth is that travel in a straight line from anywhere on the horizon will ultimately return the traveler to the same spot. We're okay with this, and we've accumulated enough frequent-flyer miles to more or less picture it. What is harder to picture is the idea that space is essentially believed to be the same way: curved, and finite but unbounded. If the technology existed to travel straight up, long enough and fast enough, an eventual return to the same spot, coming from the other side, would theoretically ensue.

The concepts of radio, television, and cell phones no longer elicit any sense of wonder. A sight or sound is transformed into a representative electromagnetic waveform that transmits at the speed of light to a receiver where it is reassembled into its original components. If you don't stop and think about this, it seems quite natural. But talking boxes and remote viewing were not natural to anyone before the twentieth century. Many shifts in existing beliefs were required, beginning with the realization that electricity and magnetism were related. They were considered separate entities until 1820, when the Danish physicist Oersted noted that a (magnetic) compass needle moved when an electric current passed nearby. During the next decades came the discoveries that these forces generated electromagnetic waves that propagated at the speed of light and that light, too, is an electromagnetic wave; that sparks generated such waves; that circuitry could be established to modulate and manipulate these waves. Now millions can watch a distant war, live, on what we call TV, and consider this normal. Or have a phone conversation between New York and Tokyo, as easily as speaking to someone in the next room, when sound itself, at the speed of sound, would take some nine hours to go that distance.

Light Amplification by the Stimulated Emission of Radiation (LASER) is a way of stimulating atoms to generate a light beam whose waves are perfectly aligned, like synchronous swimmers. Its possibility was predicted by Einstein, but its reality waited several decades until sufficient technology and ingenuity were brought to bear. Laser light creates pictures known as holograms — there's probably one on your credit card — and holograms have some unusual properties. These images are formed when a laser is split into two beams, one of which illuminates the subject and bounces off toward the film. The rest of the beam is sent back by a mirror toward the film, where the two beams cross and their interference pattern is recorded. The resulting hologram is three-dimensional, and *any* part of it can be used to regenerate an image of the entire subject (albeit, when using a relatively small part, with some loss of detail). This is not your parents' photography, and it is reminiscent of the human body, where every cell contains the DNA capable of reproducing the entire person.

Then there's Einstein's relativity. You don't need to understand it; you just need to know that, so far, it has been borne out scientifically. It dictates, among other things, that mass and energy are different forms of the same thing, and are interconvertible; that time does not progress at the same rate for everyone, everywhere; and, as Einstein himself put it: "The distinction between past, present, and future is only a stubbornly persistent illusion."[1]

Given the reality of all the above, much of what I'm going to tell you about in this book should not seem so strange. These physicians' careful observations are generally met with denial by the scientific community. But if we had always dismissed such observations, rather than trying to understand them, we would now have no TV, no lasers, no Internet, and a flat earth.

1 Einstein. The American Museum of Natural History, New York (Nov. 15, 2002–July 27, 2003).

Two

I Put a Spell on You: Witchcraft, Voodoo, and Zombies

Loosely defined, witchcraft is a ceremonial marshaling of evil (or negative) spiritual forces, a sort of flip side of prayer (which focuses positive spiritual energy). But prayer and witchcraft are not so easily or neatly polarized. People have been known to pray for the misfortunes of their enemies, and witchcraft has been used for healing and positive outcomes.

Belief in witchcraft reaches back into antiquity. Its existence was noted in Sumeria and Babylonia, in ancient Egypt and Greece, and among the Celts, centuries before Christianity. During the Roman era, laws were passed to criminalize its practice. In America, every schoolchild knows about the Salem witch trials where many innocent citizens were put to death because they were accused of casting spells and consorting with demons.

Interestingly, some scientists now believe that the fits, spells, and paranoia experienced by Salemites in 1692 were brought on by poisoning. Most of the accused witches in Salem had similar symptoms: psychosis, hallucinations, crawling sensations of the skin, twitches and spasms, headaches, vomiting, and diarrhea. These are also the symptoms of ergot poisoning. Ergot is a fungus blight that forms hallucinogenic substances in rye, and subsequently in bread. The hypothesis that the Salem witches had suffered from ergot poisoning was first published in a 1976 article in the journal *Science*, "Ergotism: The Satan Loosed in Salem?" by Linnda R. Caporael. She provides compelling evidence that the Salem witch trials coincided with a weather pattern that could easily have produced large quantities of ergot on rye, which at that time was used to make the community's bread. When the symptoms of ergot poisoning began to appear, some Salem residents, unable to explain such symptoms, jumped to supernatural conclusions.

Belief in witchcraft—in various forms and with many different names—exists today in virtually all parts of the world, including Western society, although in developing cultures it appears more widespread and visible.

Voodoo Death

Can one person, using nothing but rituals, spells, and incantations, cause another person to fall ill—or even to die? History records many such events, and scientists have struggled to find the physiology behind this deadly phenomenon. One of these scientists, Walter Bradford Cannon, is considered the father of modern neurophysiology, having elucidated the workings of the unconscious, body-regulating nervous system (autonomic) and the neurochemistry of fight-or-flight. In 1942, Cannon, a Harvard professor of medical physiology, published what he felt were reliable accounts, by outside observers, of death induced by local witch doctors or medicine men: "voodoo" deaths.

In South America, Tupinamba Indians succumbed to death apparently from fright after pronouncement and sentencing by the "medicine man." In New Zealand, a Maori woman was told she had eaten tabooed fruit. She was dead within twenty-four hours. Descriptions of such events in the Australian outback involved the slow but inexorable deterioration of the victim, usually over several days, ending in death. A Western physician working at a local mission observed no fever, pain, or signs of disease; the individual simply appeared ill and became weak, refusing food and water along the way. This fatal cascade began when the witch doctor pointed a bone—a tribally recognized form of condemnation—at the person. In one instance, the sentence was found to be reversible: After discovering that a native had been duly cursed by the witch doctor and had begun his decline, the mission physician threatened the witch doctor that his supply of food and water would be stopped if anything happened to this man. The witch doctor returned to the bedside and explained that it had been a mistake, following which the deterioration reversed almost immediately.

What these "voodoo" demises had in common was a steady downhill course, over several hours or days, proceeding much faster than the effects of deprivation of food and water alone. This differs from the classical form of death associated with intense fright or emotion, which is sudden and is generally due to a clear cardiac cause. Yet these were apparently deaths from fear. Cannon noted that a belief system was also necessary, where all members of a tribe or group hold an unwavering belief in the powers of the witch doctor, so that believing that one is doomed to die is simultaneously necessary and sufficient.

Cannon recounted similar instances from a psychiatrist's report from the Spanish Civil War regarding fatalities not from physical wounds, but from profound emotional strain. Afflicted soldiers had previously shown "lability of the sympathetic (nervous) system"—i.e., overreactive fight/flight reflexes—and "severe mental shock." Unavailability of food and water attended these deaths. Cannon tried to explain, using what was known about the nervous system's physiology at the time, what would cause this steady and terminal descent of bodily processes. Reviewing Cannon's work sixty years later in the *American Journal of Public Health*, neuroendocrinologist Esther M. Steinberg commented that today, Cannon's discoveries would never have reached publication because they are too anecdotal and unscientific—a bit paranormal, perhaps.

Modern neuroendocrinology, now more complex, adds to the plausibility of Cannon's accounts. But we still lack the precise science behind the transformation, in one to three days, of a healthy adult into a corpse, based only upon the belief that this would happen. Steinberg complimented Cannon for his courage in combining "open-mindedness and scientific rigor," and in predicting that, someday, the mechanism would be known.

Cannon clarified the role of a small area at the bottom of the brain that controls emotion and regulates bodily organs. Called the hypothalamus, it mediates everything from heart rate to digestion, automatically keeping the body, internally, on an even keel. Our hormones are also regulated here, through the adjacent pituitary gland. It was discovered independently in 1934 that packets of hormones could travel along nerve fibers (a process called neurosecretion) through the hypothalamus, meaning that electrical nerve impulses could be converted into hormones. So we now understand many of the connections between emotions, nerves, the brain, the body, and hormones, but we don't know yet how a designated sorcerer, without even the laying-on of hands, can manipulate the body's autoregulatory machinery into the ultimate meltdown.

Two Strange Cases

In "Hex Death: Voodoo Magic or Persuasion?" (1992), Nashville physician Clifton K. Meador reports two strange cases. The first, taken from the patient's doctor and nurse, occurred in 1938 and involved a sixty-year-old black man who had been ill for several weeks and had lost a lot of weight. He was hospitalized, and, despite tube-feeding and testing that revealed nothing abnormal, he deteriorated into a semi-stupor. Then his wife, after swearing the doctor to secrecy, told the following story: Four months earlier, her husband had had an argument with a local voodoo priest. During its course, the priest waved a bottle of a foul-smelling liquid near the patient's face and announced that he had been "voodooed." Along with this came an edict of secrecy, lest their loved ones get similarly cursed. Terrified, the man staggered home and began to deteriorate; seeing him near death, the wife called in a physician.

Hearing this, the physician concocted a plan (in 1938, you could do things in hospitals that wouldn't be appreciated now, like smoke cigars). The family was gathered at the bedside, and the patient was informed that the doctor had confronted and threatened the voodoo priest until the truth was told: The foul-smelling liquid contained lizard eggs, which hatched into a lizard in the patient's stomach, and was now eating him alive from within. But the doctor would rid the patient of this, and ordered a strong emetic injection (an agent that causes vomiting), which was administered by a nurse, who was "in on" the ploy. Inevitably and violently, vomiting ensued. The doctor tossed, secretly, a live green lizard into the emesis basin, the animal having been smuggled in inside his black bag. "You are now cured," he pronounced, displaying the lizard.

The patient looked suddenly dazed, then fell into a deep sleep, awakening the next morning with a hearty appetite, and was discharged from the hospital within a week. He lived ten more years. Meador heard this story in 1961; it troubled him and made no sense until he happened upon Cannon's publication.

Meador's second strange case, in 1973, concerned a man in his seventies who was known to have metastatic cancer of the esophagus, meaning that the cancer, which had begun in the esophagus, had spread to other organs—a dreadful situation. He had undergone surgery to remove the malignant esophageal tumor, as well as his stomach, to which the cancer had spread (a pouch of colon was then used to create a stomach). A scan showed that there was also cancer in the liver; he was told he had only several months to live.

When Dr. Meador first encountered the man, he was hunched up under the covers, barely able to open his eyes, and seemed unable to talk. The doctor waited, quietly, until the patient, thinking he was gone, stuck his head out from under the covers, saw the doctor, and suddenly spoke: "Go away! Leave me alone." Realizing that the man had more energy than he was letting on, the doctor arranged for intensive nursing and physical therapy intervention, forcing the patient to get out of bed and walk. This had a positive effect, as the patient gradually regained strength and appetite. He began to converse, and told the doctor a bit about his life. His first wife, his soul mate, had died suddenly and unexpectedly in an accident, after which he was heartbroken. The first symptoms of the cancer followed within six months. After the surgery, he met and married his second wife. His only wish at this juncture was to make it through Christmas (it was October); he wished to spend the holiday with his new wife and her family. They knew, he knew, his surgeon, and Dr. Meador knew that he was dying of cancer.

Because of Dr. Meador's intervention, the patient walked out of the hospital appearing healthy, a far cry from the shriveled figure originally encountered. He was well when seen at follow-up visits in the next month or two. He celebrated Christmas with his family. But he was readmitted just after New Year's, looking near death, and died within twenty-four hours. The surprise was the autopsy: one small nodule of cancer was found in the liver (the scan had erred); the disease had spread nowhere else. So he died not *from* cancer but *with* it, and from the firm belief, shared by family and physicians, that his death was inevitable.

These two cases differ from Cannon's only in the time intervals, taking months, not days. In the first instance, reversibility was demonstrated, as in Cannon's condemned man. In the second, the "witchcraft" involved was the doctors' pronouncements that the patient had only months to live—and the patient's belief in the doctors' authority. Negative thinking, it appears, is a formidable power.

Dead Men Walking

No discussion of voodoo would be complete without some mention of zombies. The word itself invokes images of a soulless body, revived from the dead. In the Hollywood version, they're evil and they don't mind eating human flesh. In Haiti, the zombie is believed to be a formerly normal person, cursed by a voodoo master (*boko*), and now devoid of any free will. The Haitian phenomenon was studied in 1997 (published in the British journal *Lancet*) by psychiatrist Roland Littlewood, who examined three such instances in detail. What these had in common was an apparent death, within three days, associated with fever. Then, years later, the individuals are found by their families, wandering in a nearby village and in a state of diminished mental and physical capacity. In two of the three cases, Littlewood was able to obtain DNA samples, which showed that the "zombie" in question was not, in fact, related to his original family; these were cases of mistaken identity, not zombification.

Littlewood noted that there is probably no single explanation for all cases. However, poisoning has long been suspected and extensively studied as a possible "cause" of zombie-hood. A 1984 report in the *Lancet* examined puffer fish toxin, which causes paralysis, sweating (which could be mistaken for fever), and lowering of body temperature and blood pressure. In other words, with no physician available to make a pronouncement, the poison victim could appear to be dead. Five zombie poisons, obtained from Haiti, were analyzed, and puffer fish toxin was found in four. Interment in rural Haiti is generally above ground, in concrete tombs which are vulnerable to break-ins, making it possible, in theory, to poison and then to recover a victim. Littlewood had interviewed two sorcerers (also known as bokos), and both used puffer fish as part of their armamentarium. These bokos noted that poisonings could be accomplished directly, or at a distance. More about impacting health from a distance will come later. For now, the Haitian zombie phenomenon can probably be scientifically understood.

Witchcraft and Lupus

Understanding of these witchcraft and voodoo hexes and healings hit a glitch in a 1981 report in the *Journal of the American Medical Association (JAMA)*, "Witchcraft and Lupus Erythematosis." Physician Richard A. Kirkpatrick described the case of a twenty-eight-year-old Philippine-American woman with a well-documented case of lupus, a multisystem disorder of unknown cause predominantly affecting young women. It is more than occasionally fatal. The patient had a high red blood cell sedimentation rate (evidence of inflammation), polyclonal gammopathy (immune system gone awry, making antibodies for no reason), and blood cells and protein in the urine, indicating leaks in the kidneys (nephritis). These, plus physical findings of an enlarged liver and lymph nodes, are characteristic of the disease, and another blood test demonstrating antibodies to the patient's own DNA confirmed the diagnosis. Lupus is known as an auto-immune disorder since it causes the body, oddly, to make antibodies to itself. Prednisone (a form of cortisone) was prescribed, and the initial results were good: the liver and lymph nodes shrank back to normal, and the kidneys stopped leaking. The dose was tapered.

Meanwhile, the patient developed hypothyroidism (low thyroid-hormone levels) and was started on thyroid replacement. The prednisone had to be increased again, as the lupus returned. She developed some well-known side effects of cortisone—swelling, a rounding of the face, and some mental changes. Her serum creatinine (a muscle-breakdown protein cleared by the kidneys) began to rise, indicating incipient renal failure. A renal biopsy was done, and showed strong evidence of auto-immune kidney damage, appropriate for lupus. High-dose, sustained prednisone, along with an immunosuppressive drug, was recommended. Instead, the patient elected to visit the remote Philippine village where she had been born.

Her family was distraught, her physicians skeptical. When she left, she was anemic, with a hemoglobin level of 9 (normal is 12–16). Her sedimentation rate was 149 (normal is 0–20), and her urine showed high levels of protein and cellular elements, known as casts, which form when cells seep into the tubules and clump together.

Three weeks later, she returned from the Philippines. She no longer had the bloated look of a cortisone-taker. She had stopped all medicines, and no signs of cortisone withdrawal, or hypothyroidism, ensued. She felt fine and refused further testing. Two years later, she delivered a healthy baby, having intermittent slight urinary protein and mild anemia during the pregnancy. These findings can be normal, and are all the more surprising since pregnancy generally exacerbates lupus.

According to the patient, the village witch doctor in the Philippines had removed a curse placed upon her by a spurned suitor. She believed her disease was cured by the removal of this "evil spirit." Kirkpatrick felt it was unlikely that the patient's lupus simply subsided, since she had biopsy-proven lupus nephritis, a high sedimentation rate, and other objective markers of disease. He ends his report with a question: "But by what mechanism did the machinations of an Asian medicine man cure active lupus nephritis, change myxedema (hypthyroidism in extremis) into euthyroidism (normalcy) and allow precipitous withdrawal from corticosteroid therapy without symptoms of adrenal insufficiency?"

Four years after her trip, she is still doing well. Kirkpatrick is nonplussed.

Witchcraft is a many-faceted thing, incorporating varying *modi operandi*; it is prevalent —and, to many people, it is real. Some of its "effects" are, in retrospect, poisonings. But some of what it purports —and has been reliably observed —to do, is presently unexplainable.

Three

Seeing Through the Mind's Eye: Psychics, Remote Viewing, and Telepathy

Here's a recent story from the newspaper: A seventeen-year-old Seattle girl named Laura Hatch vanishes. After seven unsuccessful days of searching, the sheriff's deputies assume she's run away; the family fears she's dead. She is found, however, on the eighth day, badly hurt but alive and conscious, still inside her crumpled Toyota Camry, which had crashed and tumbled two hundred feet down a ravine. How was she found? According to the paper, a volunteer searcher who said she had had several vivid dreams of a wooded area found the wrecked car in the trees. Could the girl's life have been saved by a psychic?

The Study of a Psychic

In 1975, psychologist Thelma Moss and psychiatrist Herbert Eveloff at UCLA published "A Laboratory Investigation of

Telepathy: The Study of a Psychic." The authors note that psychic phenomena have been recorded in the histories of just about every civilization, but that documentation in a scientific atmosphere has been difficult. Psychics claim that their powers cannot be switched off and on, like a radio, and may vary with surrounding conditions. So Moss and Eveloff were excited when a college junior (identified as Mr. B.) presented himself as a psychic who was willing and eager to display his gift.

First, Mr. B. underwent several hours of psychiatric examination, which determined that he had no significant psychiatric illness or delusions. Then a series of experiments was designed, which would also be applied, for comparison, to a control subject who claimed no psychic abilities. Mr. B. was going to be tested as a "receiver"; could he pick up someone else's thoughts? (He had never claimed any ability to *transmit* thoughts.) He did request that the transmitting subject—the person whose thoughts he was to receive—be someone of his choosing, since there were some people whom he felt he could work better with. Although this troubled the investigators, as it raised the possibility of collusion, it was felt that the experiment could be designed so the transmitter would not know any material in advance.

Here's how it would go down: Mr. B. would remain with one of the experiment's authors within a large institute, in a lab or office chosen at random just before starting; neither investigator nor subject would know where they would be. The young woman who was "transmitting," a high-school senior, would be taken by the other author to an undisclosed location. Neither subject/researcher pair would know where the other was.

Sessions lasted about an hour, were tape-recorded and then transcribed verbatim, looking for any matching words or concepts. Eight test sessions, and four control sessions (using the non-psychic "receiver"), were performed. The transmitter, identified as Miss K., did not know the content of the material until the session started.

As is sometimes the case in research, there were surprises. The first came just before the initial session got started. The two authors and two subjects met as a prelude to going their separate ways for the study. One author had spent the previous couple of hours with a colleague discussing ESP experiments with roulette or dice; the other had just finished playing billiards. Mr. B. would have been unaware of this, but volunteered that he was "getting something" about a roulette table and dice and something about a pool table and cue sticks on the wall. It must have seemed as if the aroma of recent conversations and activities still clung to the researchers, like the aftermath of a pungent lunch.

The session officially began when the transmitter, now separated from Mr. B., was asked to immerse her foot in ice water until it got as cold as she could bear. Then her impressions were recorded: "Cold, cold . . . feels like an amputation . . . like a ski trip in the mountains . . . once I remember I ran across an ice rink barefoot. . . ." While at the same time, but in another place, Mr. B. said: "Something to do with skiing . . . ice and water. She's going skiing this Easter. She may be talking about that now."

Later in the session a young Chinese woman, invited by the researcher and unbeknownst to Mr. B., brought in an exotic Asian dish known as a "thousand-year-old egg." Said Miss K.: "It smells like ammonia . . . it looks like something you'd find in a stagnant pond . . . like feces turned green with mold." Simultaneously, Mr. B. said: "A lime green cashmere sweater.

What a sickening color! I hate that color . . . white cups with gold trim. This is silly, it looks like China. I don't know why China would be around here."

Another surprise occurred after the session while Mr. B. and his examiner were waiting for the other pair to return. Mr. B. "picked them up," "walking out into the bright sunlight," and saw "trees breaking up the light into patches," adding: "When you look back, you can see several stories of a building." This turned out to be essentially correct, as they were at an outdoor fountain on campus, next to a building several stories high (and it's always sunny outside in southern California).

The next session brought more of the same. Miss K. was asked to punch buttons on a scratched-up metal box, while electric shocks were delivered to her left wrist, which she described as going into her hand and fingers. Mr. B. simultaneously noted "a sharp pain in my right middle finger . . . she was sitting and looking at a book or plaque . . . a metal plate with a hole in it . . . there are scratches on it . . . my left finger hurts . . . punching a button over and over. . . ."

Miss K. was unable to attend the next session due to illness, and Mr. B. offered a substitute sender, another high-school girl with whom he claimed some rapport. She was shown slides, for variety, and asked to comment. Shown a slide of a man parachuting down into the ocean, she said "A feeling of motion, the parachute is open. And white space. The ocean is white." Meanwhile, back at the (remotely located) ranch, Mr. B. perceived "an ocean . . . spray scene."

The control subject, on the other hand, was unable to "receive" anything that corresponded to the slides; his free associations showed "no recognizable correspondences," according to the authors. But then there was another surprise.

Neither of the experimental transmitters showed up for the next session. Rather than cancel, Mr. B. offered to function as transmitter, to see if the control subject could tune in to his thoughts and impressions. The researchers, already there, decided to try this from a "nothing to lose" perspective. Slides were used again; and, unexpectedly, the control—this ordinary person who was previously unable to pick up anything—was able to receive when self-proclaimed psychic Mr. B. viewed the slides. To wit: an image of Marilyn Monroe celebrating with champagne and balloons in a 1940s party background, conceptualized by Mr. B. as a "New Year's Eve party of the Roaring Twenties. High, very gay," was reported remotely by the control as ". . . like a New Year's Eve party. People celebrating." Or a picture of a dead Vietnamese soldier, riddled with bullets, was described by Mr. B. as a "Vietnam war casualty . . . mutilated, face all bloody," while the control got "Vivid war casualties . . . injured burned people . . . Vietnam war." These correspondences were as good as those obtained with the psychic as receiver, suggesting in a sense that his powers went both ways.

Mr. B.'s abilities seemed to wane with additional sessions, although he consistently did better than the control subject. Miss K. had become increasingly hassled at having to show up regularly for these; the favorable rapport that Mr. B. felt he needed may have been lacking. Looking at the earlier sessions, the authors tabulated a 54 percent success rate, based on matching words and concepts, compared with a zero success rate for the control person.

Moss and Eveloff note that Mr. B. clearly outperformed the control, and conclude that there was no choice but to consider the *possibility* that their subject had "some kind of extrasensory perception." If this seems a little wishy-washy, remember that these university-based investigators were using subjective data—comparing words instead of numbers—in a milieu where imprecision is frowned upon.

Our Psychic Spies

Now lets go to the Pentagon. The *Washington Post* broke a curious story on November 29, 1995: "Pentagon Has Spent Millions on Tips from a Trio of Psychics; CIA Wants to Shut Down Paranormal Study." Yes, this was actually in the *Washington Post.* It turns out that our government had funneled somewhere between eleven and twenty million dollars during the 1980s and '90s to support the efforts of three principal psychics working at Fort George G. Meade, Maryland, whom they consulted over two hundred times! Why would the Defense Department employ psychics? For one thing, there were several prominent members of Congress who favored this endeavor. For another, it seemed, the Russians were using psychics to spy on us. Even Saddam Hussein would eventually get into the act. In a May 5, 2003 *New Yorker* article, a confidant told the reporter that Saddam had set up a secret facility for people with special powers.

What brought the Pentagon story into the news, however, was the transfer of responsibility for the program to the CIA, and the subsequent reevaluation of the results. The CIA concluded that the psychics' information "never substantially aided U.S. national security," and felt funds should no longer be committed.

Here are some examples of what we got from our military psychics. Asked about a Soviet submarine under construction, the psychics "saw" a "very large, new submarine with 18–20 missile launch tubes and a 'large flat area' at the aft end," to be ready for launch in a hundred days. What actually happened was the sighting, 120 days later, of two Soviet subs, one with 24 launch tubes, the other with 20 and a large flat aft deck. Another time, the psychics were asked about the whereabouts of a Marine hostage, Colonel William Higgins, held in Lebanon. They conjured up a specific (real) building in a specific town in South Lebanon (names not specified in the *Post* story). This was probably correct, in that another, released hostage said that Higgins probably had been in that building at that time. In a third instance, asked about Libyan chemical weapons, the psychics predicted that a ship named *Patua* or *Potua* would arrive in Tripoli to transport chemical weapons to an eastern Libyan port. In fact, a ship named *Batato* arrived in Tripoli, loaded undetermined cargo, and then freighted it to an eastern Libyan port.

I can see how this information might not be of significant military value, as it lacks the precision of, say, an aerial photograph. (Although according to another recent *New Yorker* article, "The Image Problem," aerial photography can be very misleading.) I also see striking similarities between the readings obtained by Mr. B. in the lab and those from the Pentagon's psychics — the images are not photo quality but are well in the ballpark, albeit dreamlike. Psychics are the first to point out that their skills can be ephemeral, with great variability on different occasions. I imagine a picture going in and out of focus, or a weak station on the car radio.

Why might this be? The psychics' mood and those of their subjects seem to be a factor. Mr. B. insisted that rapport was essential. As Miss K. became increasingly annoyed at having to show up, the accuracy diminished. A boy who could "see

through walls" was brought, with his family, to Saddam's hide-
away, whereupon his powers dried right up. (Could a child
possibly have found Saddam Hussein scary?) And there are
other factors. Robert O. Becker, an orthopedist and discoverer
of some of the body's electrical and magnetic means of functioning, found that magnetic storms (which emanate from the
sun, hit the earth up to a few times a month, and affect things
like satellites and radio transmissions) adversely affect psychics' abilities.

Brain Waves

Then there are the brain's own electrical waves. The electroencephalogram (EEG) records these, usually through four pairs
of leads on the patient's scalp. The test is indispensable for evaluating epilepsy, and useful in a variety of other conditions,
including brain tumors and sleep study. The discovery of brain
waves has an interesting history. In the late 1800s, a young
German student named Hans Berger fell off his horse, only
narrowly escaping grave injury. To his astonishment, he
received a telegram from his father that very evening, asking if
he was all right, because his sister had had a "feeling" that he
might not be. Berger was so amazed by this that he changed his
major from astronomy to psychiatry and became obsessed with
finding a relationship between brain electrical activity and
human behavior. His electronic equipment was of course primitive by today's standards, but finally, in 1924, he succeeded
in recording a brain signal via metal electrodes that he stuck to
his own son's head. Thus was born an entire discipline of neurophysiology, because a girl somehow remotely viewed her
brother's brush with danger.

What might brain-wave activity have to do with telepathy? Neuroscientist Michael A. Persinger has actually studied this. Persinger worked with an artist named Ingo Swann, well known (in appropriate circles) for his psychic prowess. While Persinger has a scientist's skepticism about many paranormal reports, he accepted that Mr. Swann could "reliably draw and describe randomly selected photographs sealed in envelopes in another room." In one experiment, published in 2002, the artist was exposed to an artificial, external magnetic field that might "alter his subjective experiences"—in other words, affect his psychic function. Subsequently, his accuracy in sketching or describing distant pictures or places was ascertained, and correlated with his EEG. Persinger concludes that "remote viewing may be enhanced by complex experimentally generated magnetic fields" and that a particular EEG pattern, a 7-per-second brain wave over the back of the artist's head, tended to indicate that the descriptions were accurate.

In an earlier study, Persinger had examined many telepathic experiences and found them more frequent when the earth's own magnetic field was relatively quiet. The earth's field (which makes compasses point north, among other things) is known as the geomagnetic field, and it undergoes frequent fluctuations, imperceptible to us. Since Swann was aware that he could not obtain good visualizations from areas that were magnetically tangled, such as a maze of train tracks converging on a station, Persinger decided to test the effects of computer-generated magnetic fields on Swann's abilities.

Working with colleague S. A. Koren, color pictures containing emotional themes were clipped out of old magazines and then sealed into brown paper envelopes. These envelopes were then "immersed" in different types of computer-generated fields, to see what effect this would have on attempts by the artist to view them remotely. It turned out that if these weak magnetic fields were generated on an IBM PC-type computer running only DOS, they didn't have much effect. But if the computer was running the Windows operating system, they did interfere. Persinger believes the complexity of the fields, rather than their intensity, was the key, and the Windows-induced patterns were more complicated. He believes there are intrinsic, weak magnetic fields associated with matter, and that "our normal perceptions only extract a small fraction of the information correlated with the existence of objects." This would explain why interference from magnetic storms might also affect psychics' perceptions.

Returning to the intrinsic electromagnetic fields of the brain, there are a few more EEG studies to mention, dealing with one person's brain being able to sense EEG patterns in another's. One of the earliest studies was published in the prestigious journal *Science* in 1965. Two of fifteen pairs of identical twins were able to "synchronize" an EEG pattern, the basic alpha rhythm of 8 to 13 cycles per second that happens when you close your eyes. A twin in one room closed his eyes, generating alpha waves, which then appeared in the EEG of the second, separated twin, despite the fact that his eyes were open!

Persinger, also feeling that a genetically related brain might be more tuned to respond, studied adult siblings. In one room, the "stimulus" sibling received weak magnetic fields, externally applied to the head; in another room, the "response" sibling had the EEG recorded. With some types of magnetic stimuli to the first sibling, an EEG response in the 5–6 cycle-per-second range was noted in the second, meaning that a magnetic signal applied to one brain could affect the activity of another, at a distance. This isn't exactly reading someone's mind—brain waves reflect whole-brain processes, not individual thoughts— but it does suggest a potential interconnection, radio-style, among individuals.

Dean Radin, an electrical engineer and Ph.D. psychologist, published an interesting paper in April 2004, in the medline-indexed *Journal of Alternative and Complementary Medicine*. He chose pairs of friends and simultaneously recorded their EEGs. One friend was within a steel-walled, electromagnetically and acoustically shielded room; the other was in a dimly lit room about sixty feet away. They were asked to think about each other. The latter was periodically shown live video of the former, to reinforce such thinking, while EEG activity of both was measured. Radin found enough correlation to suggest "the presence of an unknown form of energetic or informational interaction."

In another study, in the same April 2004 issue, subjects' EEGs were tweaked by flickering lights. In five of sixty pairs, similar EEG changes could be detected in a distant person. While the percentage of successful pairs is small compared to the number of pairs tested, if this happens at all, it bears explanation. Radin, pooling earlier studies, estimates that up to fifteen percent of the pairs "show nonchance, positive EEG correlations."

So while psychics are found everywhere from the Bible to today's newspapers, it is only recently that scientific attempts are being made to electronically verify a mechanism, be it waveform or other signal, and to find what interferes with or enhances this phenomenon.

*F*our

Answered Prayers: Distant Healing and Therapeutic Touch

In the last chapter, we saw the possibilities of sensing something at a distance—brain activity, emotions, or the way a particular scene looks. Let's go one step further. We are all familiar with the concept of a force acting at a distance: Gravity pulls down, even if you're not in contact with the earth's surface; a magnet attracts nearby metal, without any contact between the two being necessary. But can a human being somehow affect others from afar?

This was the question asked by John Astin, Ph.D., in a 2000 *Annals of Internal Medicine* paper, "The Efficacy of Distant Healing," in which he reviewed twenty-three published trials examining what happens when a conscious attempt is made to benefit another person's emotional or physical well-being without making physical contact. These twenty-three were culled out because they met strict, preset inclusion criteria for high-quality research. Interventions studied included prayer, noncontact therapeutic touch, and a variety of other noncontact practices. This chapter will look at some of these trials and their outcomes.

Pray for Me

Prayer is, in Western (and other) sociological terms, mainstream and normal. It is only recently that attempts have been made to quantify some of its effects on health. Systematic use of prayer as a healing modality is common in the practice of alternative and complementary medicine, although any measurable success might be still considered paranormal, at least by conventional medical standards.

One of the first studies that made news was done during the 1980s in the coronary care unit of San Francisco General Hospital by cardiologist Randolph Byrd. Over ten months, almost four hundred patients were randomly split into a group that would be prayed for, and a group that would not. These CCU patients would not know if they were the objects of this intercessory prayer, which is a directed and purposeful praying for others. The groups were compared for twenty-six different parameters of their condition, including new problems and diagnoses and the need for medical intervention.

Three to seven intercessors, who had never met the patients, prayed for them nevertheless. They were given only their first names, diagnoses, and general condition. What's more, they prayed daily from *outside* the hospital, until the patients were discharged. The first problem with this study is the presence of what is known as a "confounder." This is something that can influence both groups in such a way as to confuse the results;

in this case, it would be friends and relatives of the patients praying for them as well. As previously noted, when there is a genetic or emotional connection between persons, it may be easier to establish a "spiritual" or "energetic" connection as well. Theoretically, if there was any effect at all of praying, family/friends' prayers could override those of well-meaning strangers.

At any rate, six of the twenty-six variables—the rates of congestive heart failure and pneumonia, the need for diuretics, antibiotics, or a respirator, and cardiac arrest—were significantly improved in the prayed-for group. "Significant" in a medical study means statistically significant—not likely to have occurred by chance (specifically, a "chance" of one out of twenty or less may be considered non-accidental). It does not necessarily imply meaningfulness in a real-life sense. For the six conditions that showed improvement, the differences were five to seven percent over the non-prayed-for group. These differences are unlikely to be accidental, but are still slim.

The bigger problem is that the other twenty illness variables—including overall mortality—were the same for both groups. Some statisticians believe it's not statistically significant when only six out of a possible twenty-six indicators change. For instance, if you roll a pair of dice, boxcars (12) or snake eyes (2) each carries a 1-in-36 chance of appearing. But twenty-six rolls will more than likely produce at least one of these improbables.

Then in 1999, researcher William S. Harris led a team at St. Luke's Hospital in Kansas City, Missouri, in an attempt to test Byrd's hypothesis. Intercessors again prayed daily, from outside the hospital, for coronary care unit patients. Again, some patients were prayed for, and some, for comparison, were not. This time, those who did the praying were only given the patient's first name, with no clinical information. Harris used a six-point scoring system to assess illness severity in a quantifiable way. He found about a 10 percent improvement in the prayed-for group, relative to the control group, with a likelihood of 1 in 25 that this was found by chance—ergo, statistically significant. But when Byrd's evaluation system was used, there were no differences found.

So here's an irony. Each study, by itself, showed that prayer helps. And each study received a fair amount of press and accolades for confirming that prayer is effective. Taken together, however, the studies are not mutually corroborative. Scientific validity requires independent confirmation, which didn't happen here. Harris nevertheless felt that his findings "support Byrd's conclusion despite the fact that we could not document an effect of prayer using his scoring method." The power of prayer is, of course, a religious belief and may not lend itself all that easily to scientific scrutiny. For all we know, its "laboratory" effects could be influenced by factors like whether the intercessors all faced in one particular direction or what the earth's geomagnetic field was doing on those particular days.

Harris cites other studies that show that regular church attendance is associated with better health. Mormon women in Utah, for instance, had much lower lung-cancer rates if their church activity level was higher. Breast and ovarian cancer were unaffected. He also made note of a study on anxiety and depression, and of one on alcoholism; these did not show a benefit of intercessory prayer.

In one study done at an arthritis/pain treatment center in

Florida published in *Southern Medical Journal* in 2000, patients with rheumatoid arthritis (a nasty affliction of joint inflammation) appeared to be helped by in-person intercessory prayer, but not by prayer from further away. In a more recent (2001) report from an outpatient facility in Miami, intercessory prayer was tried with kidney-dialysis patients. It did not make a difference, although patients who *expected* to be prayed over did better than those without this expectation. (Optimism is usually a good thing.)

Astin's review included an interesting study, which he classified as "other distant healing." It could easily have been included in the "prayer" section, as it did use an array of spiritual healers. These were chosen rather carefully, from schools and professional organizations all over the country, by word of mouth, and by reputation. For Byrd's San Francisco study, intercessors were only required to have an "active Christian life, daily devotional prayer, and active Christian fellowship with a local church." For Harris's Kansas City work, no particular religious affiliation was required, but those who would pray did need to agree with the statement "I believe in God. I believe that He is personal and is concerned with individual lives. I further believe that He is responsive to prayers for healing made on behalf of the sick."

But this 1998 endeavor, entitled "A Randomized Double-Blind Study of the Effect of Distant Healing in a Population with Advanced AIDS," essentially assembled a dream team of professional healers, requiring a minimum of five years' experience, performance of at least ten attempts of healing at a distance, and experience working with two or more people with AIDS. The team included Christian, Jewish, Native American, Buddhist, and shamanic-tradition healers, as well as graduates of secular schools of bioenergetic and meditative healing.

Psychologist Fred Sicher, the study's lead author, believed that healers do their best work when the need is greatest, so he decided to study AIDS patients who were advanced enough in the course of their disease to have had overt illness. Forty patients from the San Francisco Bay area were recruited through advertisements. Twenty would be "treated"; the other twenty would serve as controls. Neither patients, doctors, nor study personnel knew who was in the intervention group. The healers—also forty in all—were distant, all right: They were scattered all over the United States. Each was mailed photographs, first names, and current symptoms of the subjects.

Using a rotating, random healing schedule, ten different practitioners treated each subject, working an hour per day for six consecutive days. The study ran for six months. The recipients of distant healing did better. They required fewer hospitalizations (three, against twelve in the control group) and fewer physician visits, were generally less sick (graded by an illness severity score), and developed fewer AIDS-related illnesses (two instances, against twelve among controls). And they showed general mood improvement as well.

However, an indicator of prognosis—a blood count of the specific cell that the HIV virus targets, known as the CD4 lymphocyte—did not change. Six months is also not a very long time when following a prolonged, complex disease like AIDS. Nevertheless, Sicher and his colleagues were encouraged about the findings (as were Byrd and Harris about theirs) and concluded that their data "supported the possibility of a distant healing effect in AIDS." Editorializing in *The Western Journal of*

Medicine, which published the research, editor Linda Hawes Clever was less enthusiastic, feeling that the study period was relatively short and the subjects relatively few, but still felt that publication of this "provocative study" was justified "to stimulate other studies of distant healing." Independent confirmation of Sicher's results would be necessary to validate these findings.

An interesting sidenote: It's a good thing that Sicher's patients weren't being treated for warts, because "A Randomized Trial of Distant Healing for Skin Warts" in the April 2000 *American Journal of Medicine* using ten "experienced healers" found no differences in the number or size of patients' warts.

The Magic Touch

Astin also reviewed eleven trials of a healing technique known as "noncontact therapeutic touch." Hands could hover nearby, but could not make direct contact with the patient. Astin only included work that included a control or placebo group that received "mock" therapeutic touch, or, in the case of two studies where treatment was administered from behind a one-way mirror, no treatment. All reviewed trials were published between 1984 and 1998. Running these down:

- In 60 cardiovascular-unit patients where noncontact therapeutic touch was used for five minutes, there was a slight but measurable decrease in anxiety in treatment recipients.

- For 60 tension-headache patients, noncontact therapeutic touch was used for five minutes, which resulted in some pain reduction in the treated group.

- 153 patients awaiting open-heart surgery experienced the same regimen as above with no effect.

- 108 post-operative patients went through the same regimen; the treated group showed reduced need for pain medication.

- For 105 institutionalized elderly patients, noncontact touch was combined with a back rub, which the control group also received. Lower anxiety levels were noted in the treated group.

- 24 participants with experimentally inflicted puncture wounds were treated with noncontact touch from behind a one-way mirror, five minutes a day for ten days. There was more rapid healing in the treatment group. (The wounds were made by a technique known as a punch biopsy, performed after the skin is numbed. A 4-millimeter-wide plug of skin is removed, and the punch process ensures that the full thickness of skin is taken.)

- 38 participants with experimentally inflicted puncture wounds were again given therapy from behind a one-way mirror. This time the non-treated (control) group healed faster.

- 31 patients with osteoarthritis of the knee (this is a degenerative, wear-and-tear arthritis) were treated with noncontact therapeutic touch in one session per week for six weeks. No change was noted.

- 99 severe burn patients had five days' noncontact therapeutic touch for five to twenty minutes each time. The treatment group experienced less pain and anxiety, although there was no difference in pain medication usage.

- 25 participants with experimentally inflicted puncture wounds were treated with noncontact therapeutic touch. Both the treatment and control groups were treated with visualization and relaxation. There was no effect noted on either group.

- For 44 men with experimentally inflicted puncture wounds, non-contact therapeutic touch from a healer not visible to the patient was given for five minutes a day for ten days. Accelerated wound healing was noted in the intervention group.

The scorecard: Seven of the studies showed a "positive treatment effect" on at least one outcome, while three showed no effect, and one actually showed a negative effect. This is all interesting, but the hodgepodge of data so far precludes definitive conclusions.

A more recent (2001) work, "Therapeutic Touch in the Treatment of Carpal Tunnel Syndrome," was published in the *Journal of the American Board of Family Practice.* Carpal tunnel syndrome results from the pinching of a large nerve, known as the median nerve, at the wrist, causing numbness and pain. It can be diagnosed electrically by using tiny needles to measure the speed of nerve impulses across the wrist, which are slower when the nerve is squeezed. Eleven patients received "real" therapeutic touch from trained and experienced practitioners, while ten controls got a "sham" version — mimicry of the movements by untrained personnel. There was no demonstrable difference in results between the groups, but there was a surprise: Both groups improved, by the subjective measure of pain, which decreased, and by the objective measure of nerve conduction, which increased toward normal. Both groups also reported improved relaxation. In fact, for pain and nerve velocity, the "sham" patients' improvement was more significant, statistically speaking.

Why did this happen? Coincidence is possible. The authors wonder if the control patients could have inadvertently received therapeutic touch, even though the study was set up only to make it appear to patients that they might be receiving it so they would remain unbiased. Could simply going through the motions of therapeutic touch be effective? Studies like these often tend to generate more questions than answers.

A well-publicized study in the *Journal of the American Medical Association* (*JAMA*) in 1998 tested whether practitioners of therapeutic touch could detect, with their hand, the presence of another person's hand three to four inches away. This was based on the belief, central to therapeutic touch, that a "human energy field" exists which can theoretically be manipulated. Practitioners' palms faced the palms of the subjects, whom they could not see (behind a tall, opaque screen with cutouts at the base) and, as it turned out, could not reliably detect either.

Shortly after the article was published, I had occasion to try it myself. One of the nurses I worked with in a local clinic considered herself a practitioner of therapeutic touch. Her sister, also a practitioner, happened to be visiting one day, so I simulated the test conditions of the *JAMA* report, albeit crudely, and the sisters were kind enough to indulge my curiosity. Maybe my hands have been washed too many times, but they were not detectable with any consistency.

The bottom line with any treatment, of course, is whether or not it helps the patient. Thus, one can extrapolate only so much from the *JAMA* study, which did not look at disease outcomes. Astin's review of twenty-three trials of distant healing showed some positive effect for thirteen (57 percent). He notes that in the United Kingdom, there are more distant healers (about fourteen thousand) than there are practitioners of any other branch of alternative and complementary medicine.

Qi Gong

A form of traditional Chinese medicine, Qi Gong is used for distant healing through manipulation of a purported life energy known as "Qi." Garret Yount, who has a Ph.D. in molecular neurobiology, and colleagues at the California Pacific Medical Center in San Francisco recently studied the effects of external Qi Gong on the growth of human brain cells in culture plates in a laboratory. This target has the advantage of being objective — you can count cells, as opposed to asking patients if they feel better. "External" means that the Qi is directed outside the practitioner's own body: in this case, toward the growing cells.

The paper, in *BMC Complementary and Alternative Medicine,* reports on three similar experiments. The first, a "pilot" study (to see if it's worth doing a larger one), used eight trials of Qi Gong, administered toward the cells from four or more inches away, for twenty minutes. Treated cells multiplied faster than non-treated cells handled the same way. This work was done in San Francisco. Encouraged, a more formal study was set up with the same design, done in Beijing, China. This time, twenty-eight trials came up with the same result: Qi Gong made cells divide a little faster. So a third, confirmatory study was done, this time with sixty trials, also in Beijing. This time there was no difference.

It is said that research is one percent inspiration and ninety-nine percent perspiration. Add a measure of exasperation, and there you have it.

Distant healing has been around for a long, long time, and only recently have scientifically designed studies tried to evaluate it. Results are inconsistent, but worth a good look.

$\mathcal{F}$ive

Auditory Hallucinations: The Voices that Knew What They Were Talking About

Many people have heard a voice that sounded real—perhaps in a dream, or even while awake—but they could not explain where it was coming from. These are auditory hallucinations; some are fleeting and happen once in a while, while others are chronic and disrupt the normal experience of life. Some are explained by illness, injury, emotion, or disease. Others, like the case below, seem to be beyond medical explanation.

Warning Voices

In 1997, a consultant psychiatrist in London, Dr. I. O. Azuonye, reported the following case, entitled "Diagnosis Made by Hallucinatory Voices," to the *British Medical Journal:*

A full-time housewife and mother, identified by her initials, A. B., had always enjoyed good health. She had never been hospitalized and rarely sought medical attention. Born in continental Europe during the mid-1940s, she came to Britain in the late 1960s, where these events unfolded about twenty years later.

While reading quietly one evening, A. B. heard a distinct voice inside her head. The voice politely said: "Please don't be afraid. I know it must be shocking for you to hear me speaking to you like this, but this is the easiest way I could think of. My friend and I used to work at the Children's Hospital, Great Ormond Street, and we would like to help you." While A. B. knew of this hospital, she had never been there and didn't know where it was.

The voices assured her of their sincerity, even supplying some factual tidbits for A. B. to confirm (she did). But by now, the woman assumed she had gone crazy, and ran to her doctor, who of course referred her to a psychiatrist (Dr. Azuonye), which is how this all came to publication. He diagnosed a "functional hallucinatory psychosis" and offered supportive counseling and an anti-psychotic medication. Within a few weeks, the voices stopped and A. B., relieved, went on a vacation.

Although she was still taking the prescribed drug, the voices returned. This time, they told her that she needed immediate medical care, and should return to England right away. She returned, and the voices gave her an address to go to; her husband was good enough to humor her, and actually took her to the address just for reassurance. It may not have been that reassuring when it turned out to be the CAT-scanning department of a large London hospital, and that as she arrived, the voices told her to go in and have a brain CAT scan. Previously, these voices had been correct about things; this time they informed A. B. that she had a brain tumor.

She instead returned to her psychiatrist, Dr. Azuonye, who decided that the best way to reassure her was to obtain the scan. So although physical examination found absolutely no signs to suggest a tumor, the doctor ordered the test. Britain's National Health Service—their version of managed care—denied the procedure, noting the apparent absence of medical necessity. Dr. Azuonye persevered, however, and eventually the scan was allowed. The result? A brain tumor, which doctors thought to be a meningioma.

Meningiomas are neither the rarest nor the most common of cranial growths. Their cells, which arise from the brain's coverings, generally grow slowly without eating through the brain and only rarely float off to start new colonies elsewhere in the body (called metastasizing). But the space they take up squashes good brain. Removal, as soon as possible, is usually recommended. So while there were no headaches or specific neurologic abnormalities, A. B.'s neurosurgeons opted for immediate surgery. The voices told her they agreed.

Surgeons found and removed a meningioma that measured two and a half by one and a half inches—about the size of an egg. When A. B. awoke from anesthesia, the voices spoke once more: "We are pleased to have helped you. Goodbye." They never returned.

Hearing Voices

Hallucinations—of all types—are not rare. One study, done on over thirteen thousand non-institutionalized Europeans, found almost 39 percent to have experienced some sort of hallucination or imagined sensation, mostly visual, often occurring at the transition between sleep and wakefulness, and more likely when drugs, anxiety, or a history of psychiatric illness were involved.

Auditory hallucinations, the doctors' terminology for voices inside one's head, are an even more common occurrence. When a spouse dies, for instance, up to half of the surviving partners report hearing the voice, or feeling the presence, of the deceased. I once had a patient who was a minister; when I asked him how he had decided upon his career, he told me that one evening he heard the Voice of God, plain as the conversation we were having, advising him to do just that (he had had strong religious convictions to begin with). Psychiatrists consider these types of perceptions normal.

Auditory hallucinations can be amazingly real, and may take the form of music, noise, or, most often, conversation. A hospitalized fifty-seven-year-old man without mental illness, recovering from a brain abscess, was surprised to find that the folk songs he heard a boys' choir singing were not, in fact, coming from an adjacent schoolyard, nor could they be heard by anyone else. A thirty-four-year-old man with seizures arising from one of the brain's temporal lobes (the lobes closest to the temples) began to hear seemingly ordinary voices from outside his head instructing and insulting him. He attempted to tape-record them, and was shocked to find they were not on the tape. He then sought further medical attention, realizing that he had a problem.

In these two cases, a structural lesion within the brain caused the problem. Entities like tumors, infections, or bleeding can occasionally cause hallucinations, and the location of the damage may determine the type. Hearing music, for instance, is more likely with lesions near the hearing centers. But structural damage usually causes more than just hallucinations. The fifty-seven-year-old man had numbness of one side of his body, with partial paralysis. The thirty-four-year-old had seizures and abnormal electrical activity (evidenced by a brain-wave recording known as an electroencephalogram, or EEG).

Brain Tumors and Hallucinations

In 1995, neurologist C. M. Filley and colleagues reported on eight patients with brain tumors who had originally started with psychiatric symptoms. Running them down quickly:

• Patient 1 had progressive apathy, social withdrawal, and poor self-care.

• Patient 2 was apathetic and irritable and had paralysis of half of the body.

• Patient 3 suffered profound depression and ultimately developed a paralysis.

• Patient 4 had two months of auditory hallucinations (content not described) followed by memory and word-finding problems.

• Patient 5 was admitted with auditory and visual hallucinations and when examined, showed weakness of one side of the body.

• Patient 6 had disorganized thinking and flight of ideas and became manic.

• Patient 7 noted episodic fear along with numbness of the legs.

• Patient 8 had memory failure and apathy.

The authors' point was that psychiatric symptoms can sometimes be the first clue that brain tumors are present. Most mental illness, however, is not associated with brain disease (only 3 percent of institutionalized psychiatric patients are found to have intracranial tumors).

Mental Illness and Hallucinations

When mental illness is present, hallucinations are quite common. Any of the five senses can be involved (people hallucinate the feeling of insects crawling on their bodies, of strange tastes and smells, as well as visions or sounds). For whatever reason, in psychiatric patients, the most common hallucination is auditory.

Severe mental illness—psychosis—is generally divided into two primary types: disorders of thought processes (schizophrenia), and disorders of mood (depression, bipolar disorder, mania). Both are strongly hereditary. Sometimes they appear to overlap, hence the diagnostic term schizoaffective disorder (affect, as a noun, is doctorspeak for mood).

Auditory hallucinations are classically associated with schizophrenia, and occur in 60 to 90 percent of the patients. Typically these fall into three categories: 1) audible voices that restate what the patient is thinking; 2) voices that give running commentary on what the patient is doing; and 3) two or more voices arguing, usually about the patient. Often, these are accompanied by delusions. Command hallucinations—advising someone to take a particular action—have been implicated in some high-profile bizarre murders (like Son of Sam), but, when studied, were not associated with a high risk of harm to the patient or others (unlike Son of Sam). The commands are usually ignored, but are more likely to be followed when the voice is familiar, or when associated with a delusion. Whatever the format, most schizophrenics believe their auditory hallucinations are coming from the outside. A sizeable minority of patients never realizes, despite treatment, that the voices aren't real.

In a textbook example, "a 25-year-old schizophrenic farmer told of a talking tree on his property. During previous episodes he had experienced a variety of auditory hallucinations that were generally well controlled with medication. However, each time he came near this large old tree, he would hear a profound, wise voice — as if the tree were one with the earth and universe and had important guidance for him. He often came to the tree when he was troubled, seeking hallucinatory experiences."[2] This is the substance of the kinds of myths and fables that can be found in all cultures.

The Deaf Can Hear

The perception of voices is so ingrained into schizophrenia that even the deaf hear them. Dr. M. du Feu, a psychiatrist to a unit for deaf people in England, recently published a paper in a Scandinavian psychiatric journal in which sign language was used to interview schizophrenics who were born deaf. These patients, who had never heard a spoken word, were emphatic that they were hearing speech, rather than experiencing it in some other way. They described one or more voices, with content and format identical to that of the auditory hallucinations of the non-deaf. The authors make the point that the frequency and substance of schizophrenics' "voices" are about the same, deaf or not, and use words like "uncanny" and "inexplicable" to describe their findings.

Of Schizophrenics, God, and Hallucinations

Schizophrenia exists in all societies, and descriptions of its symptoms can be found throughout history. The illness afflicts

2 *Kaplan & Sadock's Comprehensive Textbook of Psychiatry*, 7th Ed. (p. 811). Philadelphia: Lippincott, Williams and Wilkins, 2000.

just under 1 percent of the world's population, with roughly equal global distribution. Its cause is obscure, but it has something to do with over-activity of dopamine, one of the brain chemicals—known as neurotransmitters—that transmit nerve impulses. Drugs that block the activity of dopamine are helpful in this disease. Some feel that schizophrenics' brains are over-wired with dopamine connections, creating paths to abnormal perceptions. People who suffer from episodes of acute schizophrenia often describe an enhancement of sensory perception. Normal people can at times experience this as well, either spontaneously, with drugs like LSD, or within religious rituals.

In a 1981 paper titled "Mystical Experience and Schizophrenia," psychiatrist Peter Buckley compared mystical experiences of non-psychotics with those of acute schizophrenia. First-person accounts are remarkably similar: heightening of perception and thinking, a sense of transport beyond the self, a slowing of time, and a feeling of communion with God. These sensations were common to both, conveying the idea that both states were enabled by enhanced reception to normal stimuli. Hallucinations occurred in both groups, but tended to be visual in the mystical group, and auditory among schizophrenics.

Auditory hallucinations also occur in other types of mental illness, though much less frequently. About twenty percent of manic patients and ten percent of depressed patients have them. Comparisons have been made between psychiatric and non-psychiatric groups. In one study, non-patients who heard voices perceived them as predominantly positive, and not scary or upsetting, as they often are in mental illness. In another study, schizophrenic hallucinators were compared to those with tinnitus (a high-pitched annoying sound in the ear, usually indicative of some sort of auditory nerve malfunction). Tinnitus is not considered hallucinatory;

it's a dysfunctional nerve firing away, creating noise. Tinnitus patients without psychiatric illness, if they hallucinated, heard music, while schizophrenics heard voices.

Getting back to A. B.'s Warning Voices . . .

The voices heard by A. B. described at the beginning of this chapter did not conform to any patterns doctors had previously run across. The eight patients with brain tumors listed earlier had overt psychiatric illness, which A.B. did not. She did not exhibit abnormal behavior, inappropriate emotion, or memory loss. Moreover, her hallucinations themselves were unlike any reported type—they were specific, goal-directed, and knowledgeable. As Dr. Azuonye put it, "this is the first and only instance I have come across in which hallucinatory voices sought to reassure the patient of their genuine interest in her welfare, offered her a specific diagnosis (there were no clinical signs that would have alerted anyone to the tumor), directed her to the type of hospital best equipped to deal with her problem, expressed pleasure that she had at last received the treatment they desired for her, bid her farewell, and thereafter disappeared."

Twelve years after her surgery, A. B. phoned Dr. Azuonye at Christmas time to wish him a happy holiday and to let him know she had done well (no voices, no tumors, no illnesses). It was then that he decided to write up the case. He wound up presenting her (in person) at a medical conference, where she was questioned about her experience. The audience could not come to any conclusion about the origin of her voices.

Some believed this to be a clear instance of telepathic communication emanating from two well-meaning people who psychically found her tumor and sought to help her.

Others theorized that A. B.'s tumor was perhaps diagnosed in her original country and that she came to Britain for free treatment under the National Health Service. But she had lived in Britain for fifteen years at the time and already was entitled to treatment, and she had also been so relieved when the voices first disappeared on medication that she celebrated with a vacation.

Another group at the conference postulated that the tumor must have caused some subtle symptoms, perhaps creating enough fear that something was wrong that she hallucinated voices reiterating this. Possibly she had unconsciously taken in information about the Children's Hospital and the CAT-scanning facility and only *thought* she had never heard of them. Maybe the voices expressing satisfaction, post-operatively, reflected her own mind's relief.

There was no conclusive evidence to support any of these theories. Suffice it to say that with unexplained phenomena, all bets may be considered "on."

Why can normal people and schizophrenics share certain experiences? How come some mentally ill, even with treatment, never come to realize that they're only hallucinating? And how did A. B.'s voices know, better than her physician, exactly what was wrong with her?

We will eventually understand all this, scientifically, and then it will be no more mysterious than invisible germs causing disease. Until then, all we know is that what happened to A. B. really did happen—Dr. Azounye, A. B., and the *British Medical Journal* didn't make it up—and there has to be an explanation for it.

$\int$ix

Animal House: Lycanthropy, or the Delusion of Being an Animal

When I graduated from medical school in 1970, homosexuality was considered a disease. Psychiatrists classified it as a personality disorder: an aberration. Treatments were administered to try to cure those so afflicted, and these therapies were famously unsuccessful. Then, in 1973, the American Psychiatric Association removed homosexuality from their *Diagnostic and Statistical Manual* (*DSM*, their all-inclusive almanac of mental illness). Being gay was no longer psychiatrically abnormal.

As a young man, and throughout my training into the early '70s, it seemed like I didn't know anyone who was gay. Homosexuality was concealed then, and apparently it could be concealed reasonably well. How things have changed. I have a gay nephew. The vice-president has a gay daughter. Such knowledge was unheard of throughout half my life.

Identity Crises

Still included in the registry of psychiatric conditions is something known as gender identity disorder, which is considered distinct from homosexuality. This is a person's strong sense, usually from childhood, that they are "trapped" in a physical body of the wrong sex, a sort of disassociation between body and soul. Some of these folks will ultimately undergo sex-change surgery (known as gender reassignment) and/or take hormones to morph their bodies in the direction of their feelings. Katherine K. Wilson, a psychologist at the Gender Identity Center of Colorado in Denver, believes that psychiatrists' only concern with gender identity disorder should be in addressing the needs of those desiring sex reassignment by medical or surgical means, and that its current classification as an abnormality provides only stigma.

Gender identity mismatch is much less common than homosexuality itself. In other words, gays experience same-sex attraction without necessarily feeling that nature gave them the wrong body. Reported cases of identity disorder find that men are affected three times as often as women. One study of boys with gender identity disorder in childhood found that the majority (in fact, two thirds: 30 of 44) became bisexually or homosexually oriented as adults. It remains to be seen if this stays classified as a psychiatric disorder, or evolves, as homosexuality did, into a mere variation of the human condition.

This chapter is about what might be called species identity disorder. Harvard Medical School psychiatrist Aaron Kulick and colleagues published, in 1990, a case report of a man who truly believed himself to be a cat. Officially, this is called lycanthropy: the delusion of being an animal. The name derives from the Greek myth of Lycaon, whom Zeus transformed into a wolf. Like homosexuality, it can be found in all cultures and throughout history, although it's decidedly less common. Kulick believes that lycanthropy is more frequent than previously thought.

The Man Who Would Be a Cat

Kulick's patient was an unmarried twenty-six-year-old man, employed full-time, who was being treated for severe depression. This problem stretched back to his freshman year at college, and included alcohol abuse, poor concentration, and disorientation. During the supervening years, a milder depression continued with intermittent severe exacerbations. By the time Kulick saw him, he couldn't eat or sleep, had no energy or motivation, was tearful, and had recently attempted suicide.

At their first meeting, the young man mentioned—by the way—that he had suspected since his childhood that he was, in fact, a cat. His youth did not sound particularly happy. He had a depressed, often bedridden, mother, and had spent many hours tied to a tree along with the family dog, whose behavior he would emulate. At age eleven, he formed some sort of relationship with the family's feline pet, and learned to "speak cat," conversing with mewing and feline gesturing. He began hanging out and hunting with the neighborhood cats, eating small prey and raw meat.

He frequently visited tigers at zoos, and communicated with them. By age seventeen, he concluded that he was some sort of tiger. More recently, he had fallen in love with a female zoo tiger, and was distraught when the animal was sold to a zoo in Asia. This event precipitated the suicide attempt.

Yet throughout his life, he had friends. In high school, he

was elected class president, and was editor of the school newspaper and yearbook. He had several extended sexual relationships with women (although he preferred the company of cats). When hospitalized, friends and colleagues visited frequently, and his interactions with them were deemed socially appropriate by hospital personnel.

But beneath it all, he considered himself a tiger with a deformed body. He outfitted himself in tiger-striped clothing, and felt more comfortable when so attired. He sported sideburns, moustache, and beard, all bushy but well groomed, and kept his nails long; he maintained a rather feline appearance.

He had enough connection to the reality of contemporary American society to conceal his "true" identity. At seventeen, he did confide in a few close friends and psychiatrists. He often required formal psychiatric care, due to depression and perhaps to the stresses of living what he saw as a lie. There was mental illness in his family: a grandfather and cousin had committed suicide; two aunts had died in psychiatric institutions. He himself had required four psychiatric hospitalizations beginning at age nineteen, three of which were at Kulick's facility.

During these breakdowns, he sometimes hallucinated a tiger companion; at other times he became non-functional and growled and crouched in feline positions, sometimes for several days. In lighter moments, he bemoaned his physical, non-cat body but maintained his fundamental obsession. Otherwise, thought processes and perceptions were usually intact.

And he received treatment. Lots of it. Smorgasboards of antidepressants, tranquilizers, and mood stabilizers. Electroconvulsive shock therapy. Psychotherapy. While these alleviated the depression, they never took away the central theme of his life, that he had been born a cat. At the time the paper appeared in *The Journal of Nervous and Mental Disease,* he was on several medications, sharing an apartment with two friends, and working and functioning well. What impressed Kulick was the stubborn resistance of his patient's basic delusion to treatment.

More Cases

Kulick's colleague, Paul Keck, had been the lead author of a 1998 study, "Lycanthropy: Alive and Well in the 20th Century." Keck *et al.* collected, from memory, twelve cases from McLean Hospital in Boston over the previous twelve years of patients who claimed to be, or acted like, animals. These were psychiatric inpatients, and their lycanthropic behavior generally occurred within the context of acute or chronic mental illness. Keck believed that the nature of these patients' psychiatric illnesses was no different from those of the hospital population as a whole. That is, no specific psychiatric syndrome could be expected to include, or exclude, lycanthropy.

Five previously reported cases were reviewed in the paper: three were wolves, two were dogs. All had remitted (i.e., lost the animal alter ego) with therapy, which was predominantly drug treatment. Keck's twelve new cases included six who identified themselves as canines (wolves or dogs), two who believed they were cats, another a gerbil, yet another a bird, and two who did not embody a specific animal but exhibited feral behavior, like growling, crawling, hooting, or howling. Treatment accomplished remission in seven of them, partial remission in three, and not much in two. In clinical parlance, those two would be known as refractory to treatment.

As mentioned, there was nothing distinctive about these

patients' psychiatric diagnoses (other than the lycanthropy). Overall prognosis did not seem to be related to animal identification syndromes. These patients were medically and neurologically unremarkable, meaning that neither physical examination nor laboratory studies turned up specific abnormalities.

Kulick and his co-authors are struck by the fact that lycanthropy cases, although rare, can still be found, and that many such individuals may go undetected or undiagnosed. Co-workers and acquaintances of the "cat-man" may have found him a little odd, but likely had no idea what was really going on inside him.

His burden of deceit is in many ways a consequence of the society and times he lives in. Believing oneself to be an animal, or being perceived as one by others, is a big negative. But in some cultures, lycanthropy may not be a bad thing. Kulick's paper refers to accounts of a Mexican Yaqui Indian shaman who metamorphosed into an animal via ritualistic use of psychedelic drugs. Also described is the Bororo tribe of Brazil, whose shamans experienced spirit possession, and whose transformations into native animals enhanced their healing powers. Some African shamans use a healing process in which the patient becomes an animal who is unable to suffer the human's disease. So in another time and place, the tiger/man could have been someone sought out by his contemporaries for medical help.

The particular animal one becomes is also era- and culture-dependent. Lycos is Greek for wolf, and technically the wolf-man is the archetype. In Europe, the wolf, with its aura of fear, respect, admiration, and power, has been the traditional species identification, although in modern times the dog is becoming more popular. In Africa and Southeast Asia, the hyena, tiger, crocodile, or shark may be chosen.

Fox Possession

In Japan, where the fox occupies a special place in folklore, it may become the lycanthropic beast of burden. In "The Interpretations of Fox Possession: Illness as Metaphor," published in *Culture, Medicine and Psychiatry* in 1991, sociologist Matsuoka Etsuko describes the case of a woman who believes herself possessed by a fox spirit. In Japanese culture, the fox is considered by some to be a deity, and it occasionally becomes an object of worship. The fox is also considered a trickster that can change into a young woman and bend people to its will.

Shamanistic practitioners still exist in Japan, although they are somewhat hidden. They may be consulted when one suffers from a condition that mainstream physicians can't remedy. Fox-possession would be such a condition, and the woman, known as Michiko, sought advice from a shaman in 1983. The author was studying the shaman and her cult group when Michiko, then age forty-three, presented herself with a complaint of hearing voices and sounds, which she attributed to foxes. When asked by the researcher how she knew the spirits were foxes, she claimed to have seen one, "very small because it was a spirit."

Michiko had always had some acceptance of a spirit world (she had tried to contact her dead parents through a medium). She also had a relationship with Japan's mental health system, having been hospitalized at one time for seven months, to no avail. She originally did not consider spirit possession to be her problem, but sought out shamans after the hospitalization, realizing that conventional medicine hadn't helped.

At first, these shamans didn't help either, but Michiko kept trying and ultimately found the healer whom Etsuko was researching. After several months, however, the fox-possessed patient felt herself to be evolving shamanistic powers, which created a conflict and jealously in her relationship with this shaman. After about a year, she stopped going. Dr. Etsuko followed the patient until 1988. By then, she seemed calmer but still believed in the world of spirits and still felt herself to be possessed, although no longer by a fox.

Unlike the cases previously discussed, Michiko did not feel she actually *was* a fox, and didn't act like one. She simply believed she was somehow taken over by the spirit of a fox, saw spirit foxes, and at times conversed with them. The parallels with the other lycanthropes, including the shamanistic transformation, are obvious if not identical. To the sociologist author, the fox is a metaphor that enables the patient to understand and explain her symptoms as something concrete and authentic.

Etsuko also discusses common characteristics of spirit possessions in Japanese and other cultures. Spirits are perceived as capricious, demanding, vengeful, and potentially dangerous. They can adversely affect health and behavior. They must be dealt with: expelled, obeyed, or befriended.

Past and Present

Accounts of human/animal flips go back to the Bible. In the book of Daniel (4:32–33), God punishes Babylonian King Nebuchadnezzar by changing him into an ox. Greek mythology as well as ancient Greek medical treatises describe the condition. Then there's the werewolf (literally man-wolf) legend of European folklore. During the Middle Ages, the going belief was that this connoted Satanic influence or demonic possession. Recent medical theories include poisonings with hallucinogenics, either accidental (like the Salem witches' ergot ingestion) or purposeful. Another theory relates werewolfery to a rare, congenital disease known as erythopoetic porphyria, where the skin darkens and facial hair grows effusively, perhaps giving one a lupine appearance and a tendency, via embarrassment, to prefer darkness. Still another speculation posited rabies as a cause. Some feel Medieval "wolf-children" may have suffered from autism.

Today, lycanthropy is considered a form of psychiatric illness. Unlike homosexuality, I don't see it being declassified any time soon. Four to ten percent of the American population identify themselves as gay, depending on the criteria used, but extensive studies from genetic, environmental, hormonal, and brain-scanning perspectives have provided no consistent data as to how or why homosexuality happens. Gender identity disorder, seen in a much smaller percentage of the population and still on the books as psychiatrically abnormal, must be caused by *something*, but current paradigms do not seem to be homing in on the answer. How does someone get it into their head, all their lives, that physically they are of the incorrect sex?

Even more puzzling, how does someone come to believe they are of an entirely different species? Lycanthropy, which may or may not share some possible avenue of causation with gender identity disorder, also represents a bad fit of body and soul. How does this happen? Even if the delusion, through psychiatric treatment, can be stuffed away out of consciousness, where did it come from? How can a man, throughout his life and despite therapy, believe he is truly a cat? And how many more like him are concealed within our midst?

$\mathcal{S}$even

Intimate Demons: Cacodemonomania, or Sex with the Devil; Ghost Possession

Possessed by the devil. That's a concept that goes back to antiquity and continues to resurface, in all eras and cultures. Nowadays, the "possessed" are psychiatric patients, and most of them can be understood or even righted within the context of what we know about mental illness. But now and then, odd cases pop up.

A Case of . . .

Consider a report of a British woman, published in 1987 in the journal *Psychiatry*, under the cacophonous title "Cacodemonomania," which is the belief that one is possessed by a demon. In this woman's case, she experienced nothing less than having had sex with the devil. Psychiatrists Paula Salmons and David Clarke detailed this story of a married teacher known as Mrs. A.

Mrs. A.'s history prior to her affliction was what we call unremarkable. She was adopted; infancy and childhood passed without incident or surprise. She completed her schooling and became a teacher. At twenty-three, she married another teacher; they would have three children.

Her problems began ten years later. She became tired and depressed, and felt unconnected to the events of her life. To the psychiatrists, she appeared to be suffering from an atypical depression plus depersonalization (the technical term for "detached"). She was put on medication, but symptoms of unreality and depression continued for the next two years.

At about this time, Mrs. A. commenced having strange hallucinatory occurrences. Lying in bed with her husband, she thought he had changed physically. Not the usual thing, like developing a paunch, but rather growing extra eyes and limbs and skin that felt scaly to touch. This only lasted a few minutes, but in its aftermath came persistent mood swings with well-punctuated highs and lows. Once, while taking a bath, she was sure she was shedding large chunks of her skin, and even saw them clogging the drain.

She was still on medication while this occurred, but then she became pregnant with her third child, so all drugs were discontinued. The pregnancy passed uneventfully. A normal baby girl came into the world, and the situation remained copacetic until the child was four months old. Then, one day, Mrs. A. suddenly became aware of an intense odor, which she likened to that of a newborn baby. Her own baby was in another room at the time, presumably out of smelling distance. The mother felt that her baby's skin was peeling off in a bizarre way. She saw these peelings wrapped around the refrigerator.

Some months later, during a reading of the New Testament in a bible class, Mrs. A. got a distinct sense that her own god was different from the god experienced by others. A "force" inside her suggested that there were pleasures available well beyond anything she could experience through reading the Bible. Over the next two years, this woman believed she had sexual intercourse with this force, "as with a man." The episodes included a feeling of penetration resulting in orgasm, sometimes pleasurable, often not. Sex with her own husband became unpleasant and ultimately repulsive to her.

Mrs. A. held orthodox Christian religious beliefs. Her minister, whom she consulted, believed she was possessed by a "malevolent force" that was responsible for her behavior and general misery, and that successful treatment must be spiritual rather than medical. Despite his recommendation, she was shortly admitted to a psychiatric hospital.

The doctors found her to be neat and well dressed. She appeared and behaved appropriately, and established rapport with the staff. But it was difficult for her to detail her "sexual" experiences, and she was a bit evasive on this point. Nevertheless, her emotional mood was normal, although slightly cool. She showed no evidence of any big-time psychiatric illness (or psychosis, as we call it); her thought processes and understandings of things were intact. Physical examination and routine bloodwork were normal. An electroencephalogram (brain-wave test) at first found a minor abnormality, but subsequent testing was normal. A brain CAT scan was also of no clinical significance. Mrs. A. ultimately declined further medical treatment.

The psychiatrists did not know quite what to make of Mrs. A.'s case. No single psychiatric diagnosis would explain all her symptoms. Delusions and hallucinations are common in the psychosis known as schizophrenia, but this patient lacked other features of this condition. There were no biological features of depression (these might include problems eating or sleeping, unusual fatigue, or inability to concentrate). There was no physical illness found. The authors feel that this is a rare case, but one that is seen occasionally: no single discipline (like psychiatry) adequately explains it. The doctors conclude that "A broader perspective is required," which encompasses the patient's symptoms, subculture, and spiritual life.

My Father, the Devil

Others have come to that conclusion. Psychiatrists Eric Schendel and Ronald Kourany, in a 1980 paper, "Cacodemonomania and Exorcism in Children," reviewed the cases of five children, aged seven through seventeen, whose families thought they were demon-possessed. All were seen at the Vanderbilt University Medical Center in Nashville, Tennessee.

- An eleven-year-old white boy was brought in because of rebelliousness, school problems, and difficulty getting along with his peers and siblings. His parents had divorced when he was five, and he rarely saw his father. His mother felt that his problems had started when he was seven, after an accident that, she felt, made his legs grow unequally. She sought out faith healers and saw her son's short leg "grow out before her eyes." At ten, a religious group attempted an exorcism, which drove the boy "berserk" but reinforced the mother's belief that her son was possessed by demons. The doctors found the child to be alert, friendly, and well behaved, with normal speech and thought processes. A tinge of depression and low self-esteem was noted. They diagnosed adjustment reaction, depressive type, which means the same in medicalese or English, and recommended outpatient psychotherapy. After nine sessions, however, the mother and boy left town.

• A seven-year-old white boy was admitted to the psychiatric unit because of aggressive behavior and fighting. His parents had divorced during his infancy; the mother remarried but had mental and marital problems herself. She had tried "everything" to set the child right, without success. A month before the admission, her church members informed her that demons had "taken possession" of the boy and needed to be "driven out." A church service was organized to do just that, but despite some dramatics and the boy's feeling that the demons had left, his behavioral problems worsened. On examination at the hospital, he was alert, cooperative, and clear-thinking. He showed a wide range of emotion and had difficulty talking about his relationship with his mother. There was a sense of poor impulse control. He was diagnosed with possible severe anxiety reaction, and showed some improvement during the hospitalization, but his mother signed him out against medical advice.

• An eleven-year-old white girl became a psychiatric inpatient due to headaches, violent outbursts, and difficulty getting along with her peers. Her parents had divorced when she was two, and she had only sporadic contact with her father. This was a girl who could get quite violent. She claimed to be aware of what she was doing, but was unable to control herself, that "someone else" was commandeering her body. Her family decided she was devil-possessed, and she agreed. She was prayed over by her church and felt better afterward for a while. Upon hospital admission, she was alert, intelligent, and articulate. She seemed older than eleven and a bit seductive. Thought processes were normal. Her diagnosis, tentatively, was conversion reaction, meaning that she converted mental conflicts into physical symptoms. She did well, but her mother had her discharged against medical advice.

• A seventeen-year-old black girl, an outpatient, believed she was possessed by the devil and that she was seeing the spirit of her dead mother. For the previous three years, she had been paranoid and had been hearing things. Her mother had been murdered when she was twelve, and thereafter she lived with her grandparents and reported sexual molestation by other members of the family. The extended family believed in witchcraft and other supernatural phenomena. Examination found her emotionless, having delusions, and with scrambled thought processes. She was diagnosed with paranoid schizophrenia, the most common type of schizophrenic psychosis. A strong tranquilizer was prescribed, but the teenager never returned.

- A thirteen-year-old white boy was admitted to the inpatient unit because he was withdrawn and exhibited bizarre behavior. He believed demons had entered his body two years earlier, and at times controlled him and rendered him violent. His parents had divorced when he was four years old, and his mother, with whom he lived, had been diagnosed as schizophrenic. The family subscribed to a number of occult beliefs, and there were frequent conversations about demons and spirits. To the physicians he was aloof and delusional, and he heard and saw things. He was diagnosed as schizophrenic and started on medication, but was removed from the hospital by his mother, against medical advice.

These five cases have a lot in common. All came from families with connections to the occult. All had lost contact with a parent through death or divorce. Freud had described a case where he felt the devil was used as an unconscious replacement for a man's dead father. Psychiatrist James Bozzuto noted that the book and movie *The Exorcist* described the possession of a girl who had lost a father, and thought such states might represent a defense mechanism against parental loss. In any event, none of these families had much enthusiasm for "modern medicine," and they all turned away from it quickly. None of the five patients above stayed around to be treated by psychiatrists. Doctors Schendel and Kourany seize upon the point that any serious attempt at treatment here must include the families' cultural beliefs and involve a team approach, even involving "an empathetic yet enlightened religious figure from the patient's faith." This is reminiscent of the "broader perspective" needed to understand Mrs. A.'s illness at this chapter's beginning.

Mrs. A., being adopted, could also be seen as having lost parents. And, like the children above, her worldview included the concept of evil spirit possession (her minister's view was that she was possessed by a "malevolent force"). As noted in the chapter on witchcraft, in order to be susceptible to such malevolence, a person has to believe, and has to exist within a community of believers. Physicians who understand this may be able to intercede, like the one who made the South American Indian witch doctor reverse his curse, or the one who put a live lizard in his black bag to be produced at the bedside to convince a hospital patient that he was cured.

I Am Not Myself

Psychiatrists call it a dissociative disorder when someone seems to separate (i.e., dissociate) from who they actually are. As *Kaplan & Sadock's Concise Textbook of Clinical Psychiatry*, 2nd ed., 2004, puts it, they've "lost the sense of having one consciousness. They feel as though they either have no identity, are confused about who they are, or experience multiple identities." Subclassifications of dissociative disorder include trance disorder, and its correlate, possession trance. These are "disturbances in . . . consciousness, identity, or memory that are indigenous to particular locations and cultures." An altered state of consciousness defines these conditions, and may involve hallucinations or feelings of being taken over by an alien, controlling spirit. There is often no memory of the episode.

The five patients above might qualify. Their belief systems allowed for demons or the devil. Their perceptions and actions appeared not to be under their control. Sometimes the explanation is simple. In an earlier edition of the *Textbook,* an example is given where a husband's guilt over an extramarital liaison led him to believe that he was devil-possessed. Therapy, using hypnosis and directed at the underlying cause, was successful.

But sometimes things are not so straightforward. The next patient you'll meet came from a culture where ghost possession was accepted. If his case sounds strange, psychiatry's bottom line, according to the 2004 *Textbook,* is that "possession and trance states are curious and imperfectly understood forms of dissociation." I'd have to agree.

Comes a Ghost

London psychiatrist Anthony Hale reported a case of ghost possession in 1994 in the *British Journal of Psychiatry.* The patient was a well-educated and intelligent young man of south Asian Hindu descent. He seemed to have settled into a life of petty crime, and his story emerged during a prison stint. Put simply, he felt that his bad behavior was caused by a ghost.

His family had come to England when he was six; he was Westernized in his appearance and manner. The problems began at age eleven, at a family gathering where an aunt, jealous of his family's success, fed him "cursed rice," which made him susceptible to spirit possession. Subsequently he was at times taken over by the ghost of an old woman, whom he did not recognize, and who made him do malicious things, while his normal "self" could not react.

He could actually see the possession coming: A visible fog came drifting toward him. The fog would settle on his chest, making it hard for him to breathe, and then would enter his body through his nose and mouth, as he retched and wheezed in resistance. Then his entire body, even his voice, was under ghost-control.

These interludes lasted anywhere from half an hour to several days, and he could remember them. He retained awareness of his surroundings and his emotions (usually fear, anger, and guilt), but everything looked hazy, and he had no control over his bodily actions. The voice of the ghost sometimes commanded him to do things; at other times he could hear this voice commenting to unseeable others. He felt that the ghost could hear him even when he wasn't in its power.

Upon medical examination, the man did not appear to be having panic attacks, nor was he hyperventilating. There were no stresses in his life that precipitated these episodes. He experienced a feeling of warmth, but had no fever. Routine blood testing, physical examination, and urine screening for illicit drugs were negative. CAT scan and electroencephalogram were normal.

The young fellow said that he gained nothing from his sallies into crime: He didn't need money; he derived no excitement. His family were well-to-do professionals, and he knew how hurtful his behavior was to them (although the jealous aunt rather enjoyed it). In desperation, his family sent him to holy places in India where exorcisms were performed, first in the Hindu tradition, then Moslem, and finally Christian, all of which were unsuccessful.

This would have been a garden-variety "possession" case — tagged with a psychiatric diagnosis or two by Western physicians, while taken literally by members of the patient's own culture — except for one thing: The authors of this paper were "disturbed" by a phone call from the prison chaplain who said that *he* also had seen the ghost. Not only did the chaplain see the ghost, but he watched as a cloud with a face (a face that "alarmingly," according to the authors, fit the description of the old woman that they had obtained from the patient) descended upon the prisoner. Even other prisoners saw it, and found it rather frightening! The chaplain denied any prior knowledge of this apparition.

So the doctors were left with a patient they considered to be suffering from a dissociative state or paranoid schizophrenia, four priests (the three in India plus the chaplain) from three religions who doubted that all this was merely delusional, and a law-enforcement system that knew a malingerer when it saw one.

Ironically, this story has a happy ending, at least for the several months during which the young man was followed up. Exorcisms having failed, he was medicated with a strong antischizophrenic tranquilizer, and his problems ceased.

The young man was not alone in believing that he was being ghost-guided at times. Ghost-inflicted illnesses are part of the subculture in some areas of Hindu India, and are interwoven with Hindu beliefs. Anthropologists Ruth and Stanley Freed traveled to a village in northern India to study this, and found a well-structured belief system that allowed for such maladies. In it, a person's soul at the time of death becomes a ghost, briefly, that may pass on naturally, or wander unnaturally, still a ghost. The more painful or untimely the death has been, the more likely it is to produce a wandering ghost. (Western cultures frequently foster the same beliefs — every trick-or-treater knows that the more horrific the death of a house's inhabitants, the more likely it is to be "haunted.")

Two types of afflictions result: ghost illness, with fever, pain, difficulty breathing, and, occasionally, delirium; and ghost possession, which is pretty much what the educated London man experienced, except that in a typical case, there is no memory of what happens while under the influence. The Freeds substantiated thirty-eight cases, and found men and women to be equally affected, regardless of caste.

One of the more common hauntings occurred when a first wife died unhappily and before her allotted time, returning as a ghost to terrorize . . . the second wife. (I know some Western women who might consider this justified, if not plausible.) At any rate, to the villagers, the solution to all these evil enchantments was exorcism, at times combined with conventional medicine, like antibiotics. Whatever works. This is the conclusion that most conventional physicians who treat these patients have come to: There is no one way to successfully deal with those "possessed"; you need a multidisciplinary team.

A check on exorcism in the medical literature, however, turns up a number of fatal, if well-intended, attempts. It's possible that these get written up and published faster than the (less credible) success stories, but the bottom line is: Don't try this at home.

And "the devil made me do it" is still not a valid legal defense.

$\mathcal{E}$ight

Dying Right on Time:
Self-Predicted Death

For many years, I worked at a county-sponsored general medical clinic. The clientele were mostly lower-middle-class/working-class families, and one day when I came to work I learned that a rather strange thing had happened to one of our patients. He had died over the weekend, which was not in itself unusual, especially as he was eighty years old. But the news of *how* this happened spread a wave of goosebumps through the employees of our health center.

The Banker's Last Withdrawal

The patient had come to the United States from his native Italy as a young man. From a job as a bank teller, he gradually worked his way up to vice-president and, in due course, ultimately retired. He had raised a family, was an accomplished musician, and spoke several languages. He and his wife often spent time in their Florida home; otherwise they stayed with their son on Long Island, which is how we knew him. The son, who was kind enough to speak with me, was an eyewitness to the event and supplied me with these details.

The plan was for the son to fly down to Florida to pick up his parents so they could all drive back in the parents' car to New York, where they would be staying at the son's home for a while. The car would then become the son's; the father was going buy a new one. The older man's health was not great—he had had a stroke two years earlier that left him unable to play his treasured mandolin—but he was in stable condition, lived independently with his wife, and was mentally clear. On arrival in Florida, the son thought his father didn't look well, and he suggested that they fly back, rather than drive; but the father insisted on driving as originally planned. As they left for the drive north, it was the son's impression that his father, last to leave the apartment, paused at the door as if locking it thoughtfully.

After they arrived in New York, for some reason the older man did not want to shop for new cars, as they had planned. Then, on a Sunday afternoon, ten days into the visit, he sat down in the kitchen and summoned his family. He had his wife prepare him ravioli (his favorite meal), and appeared to eat heartily. He even had wine and dessert. After that, he sent his seven-year-old granddaughter outside to play. Sitting at the table with his wife, his son, and his son's girlfriend, he began apportioning his possessions. The family was somewhere between puzzled and horrified. It was not this former bank executive's nature to be impulsive. There seemed to be no necessity for doing any of this now, as he didn't appear particularly ill. He even insisted on signing the papers on the car, transferring ownership to his son. "Take good care of your mother," he told him.

Then he closed his eyes and died, still sitting in his chair at the kitchen table.

The ambulance came within minutes, but on-the-spot cardiopulmonary resuscitation failed, as did attempts at a nearby hospital. The assumption was that this must have been a "massive coronary," but no autopsy was done. He had simply closed his eyes and died.

After the funeral, the son went back to Florida and discovered that his father had transferred the title to his stocks and bonds, and had put all his affairs in order. It was as if he had died deliberately.

I wrote up this interesting case, and my report was published in *Psychology Today* in 1983. After the publication appeared, I received a number of interesting letters, as well as commentaries from friends, co-workers, and patients. Well-arranged deaths are apparently not that rare. I was told of a doctor's mother-in-law who died peacefully in her sleep after having made all the possible arrangements her demise would require, including selling her house. A letter from a woman in Seattle told of her father's death: A week before it, he had made sure his wife knew where the safe-deposit box key and all important papers were; he sold his tools and made sure all affairs were in order. Then he died of a "massive coronary," although there was no mention of chest pain in the week preceding. In another letter, a fifty-five-year-old woman wrote me her essential life story, which included the loss of a loved one five years earlier which had undercut her very will to live; she also mentioned some unfinished work she still needed to complete. She said it was easier to "let go" than to finish the work, but she would nevertheless wait until all was done, about a year later, "to turn off her life naturally," emphasizing "no suicide." (Unfortunately, I don't know what ultimately happened to her.)

The Spartan Buys a Headstone

A tale similar to the one I reported was published in *Life* magazine, still in its heyday in 1960 ("The Man Who Died on Time"). This fellow, who was seventy-seven, had emigrated from Greece many years earlier and lived first in New York City, and then in a small Ohio town. He was a big, strong man — "a Spartan," as he referred to himself — and was also a bit of an eccentric. For example, he stopped at green lights and drove through red ones. He never had a wife or children, had no close friends, and his nearest relatives were a sister and a nephew living in Michigan.

He owned a shoeshine parlor, which he closed when he was seventy, after which he became a recluse. A year and a half before his death, he purchased a cemetery plot and proceeded to visit it weekly, as if it were a second home. He would bring gardening tools and make sure the plot was perfectly landscaped, even adding a potted geranium on Memorial Day. He told cemetery workmen (who may have been wondering why someone was visiting his own grave) that he wanted to enjoy the flowers now; he wouldn't be able to see them after he was gone.

Continuing this saga, he purchased a vault and casket from a funeral home, and had the home's undertaker help him write his own obituary; he couldn't understand why the newspaper wouldn't run it until *after* he died. He bought a headstone along with two Japanese yew trees to be planted on either side, and he discussed their care and feeding with cemetery workers during his regular visits. He ordered flowers for his own funeral.

Then, paradoxically, he went to a local hospital for a checkup (as I said, he was eccentric). Of course, he got a clean bill of health. Shortly afterward, he called his nephew and asked him to bring his wife and three children, as well as the man's sister, down from Michigan for an "important" visit. On their arrival, he showed his nephew three envelopes containing money, one for each of the nephew's three children. The nephew was sufficiently perplexed to call the hospital where his uncle had just been checked over to confirm the "clean bill" (which they did).

They all went out to eat, and on the way back to the uncle's apartment he had them stop at the cemetery to see the headstone, already inscribed. As the nephew's anxiety and confusion increased, the older man simply became more cheerful. When they returned to his apartment, he handed the nephew his will, made sure he knew which pocket the envelopes for the children were in, and emptied the pantry, packing the goods into boxes for his nephew's wife. Then he gave out some remaining possessions, and when the nephew protested that his uncle needed these things for himself, the old Spartan replied, "No, boy, I don't need anything any more."

Then he fell down dead. The doctor arrived within minutes, and said it must have been a heart attack. Nothing needed to be done. All the arrangements had been made.

The banker and the Spartan told no one of their impending ends; they simply went about their business as if it were a done deal. No autopsies or official medical diagnoses were available. This next case, reported in the British journal *Lancet* in 1980, concerns a 40-year-old Massachusetts housewife who spent five days in the hospital with an evolving heart attack, under close medical scrutiny.

The Mother and the Prophecy

This mother of five had an elevated cholesterol level, most likely hereditary, for which she was on medication. She began having chest pains but continued her usual activities, including tennis, for three days. Then she sought medical attention and was promptly admitted to a hospital. Although she appeared comfortable at the time, and complained of only mild pain, her electrocardiogram (EKG) showed signs of acute cardiac damage.

The next day, the patient announced to her physicians, her nurses, and her clergyman that she would die three days hence, on May 28, the anniversary of her mother's death. She repeated this prediction to anyone who came by her bedside, over their protestations. During this time, her EKG's reflected the progressive changes of an active heart attack, and blood tests confirmed this. By May 27 she appeared peaceful, detached from the seriousness of her illness. Early the next morning, as she predicted, she died. Her heart simply gave out (rapidly progressive cardiogenic shock, in the vernacular).

This time an autopsy *was* performed, and it confirmed what the pre-mortem tests had shown: an extensive myocardial infarction. The only curious thing was that the coronary arteries—the blood vessels that feed the heart muscle itself—were wide open. Most heart attacks occur because one or more of these vessels becomes occluded. But in a small number of cases, a coronary transpires without any evidence of blockage. Spasm of these arteries, occurring for reasons unknown, can be sufficient to shut them down. Spasms cannot be predicted. How she could have called her death three days in advance, or have had any control over it, is a complete mystery.

"Self-Predicted Fatal Myocardial Infarction in the Absence of Coronary Artery Disease" was how the *Lancet* piece was entitled, and its author, Dr. Robert Carey, wonders if coronary artery spasm could have been responsible, and if such spasms might be a common feature of unexplained death, particularly under emotional stress.

Stress and Death

The fact that people die suddenly in situations of extreme fear or emotion was addressed in a 1971 paper by psychiatrist George Engel of the University of Rochester. "Sudden and Rapid Death During Psychological Stress—Folklore or Folk Wisdom?" examines the concept of sudden death from emotional shock. While it is virtually common knowledge among physicians and lay people alike that this occurs (almost everyone has an anecdote), Engel tried to examine the phenomenon systematically. He collected, over a six-year period, newspaper accounts of 170 people who succumbed suddenly after an emotional trauma. Suicides were excluded, and most of these deaths occurred within an hour of the reported trauma. News releases were used because of the impossibility of obtaining relevant data on sufficient numbers of people in any other way.

Throughout history, there are many recorded instances of immediate death from fright or emotion. In the Bible, for instance, Ananias falls down dead when Peter tells him "You have not lied to man but to God" (Acts 5). Now Engel could examine this process, through his series of cases reported in newspapers, for the details. He was able to divide these into eight "causes," listed here in decreasing order of frequency:

- **Impending danger.** This was the single most common cause, and included natural disasters, like earthquakes or storms, as well as muggings, fighting fires, and courtroom or police questioning. This group included a three-year-old who died during a severe rainstorm and a four-year-old who expired while having teeth pulled. There were even three casualties recorded during the viewing of particularly gory scenes on TV.

- **The collapse or sudden death of a close person.** In some of the cases attributed to a sudden loss, heart failure was implicated. In the case of the wife of the owner of the motel where Martin Luther King was assassinated, a brain hemorrhage felled her the same day.

- **During a time of acute grieving (within sixteen days).** In this category, Engel cited a twenty-seven-year-old army captain who died after leading the ceremonial troops at the funeral of assassinated President John F. Kennedy.

- **The threat of loss of a close person.** Of the sixteen people who experienced the threat of loss, eleven deaths were sudden and dramatic, attributed to heart attacks, although there was no medical confirmation. The other five were reactions to the burden of prolonged illness in a family member, which the author feels is a not-uncommon precipitant.

- **Following a dangerous event.** Instances of demise *after* the danger has passed may reflect the high levels of adrenalin and related substances still circulating in the bloodstream. In an unrelated study of exercise, looking at why cardiac deaths sometimes occur in an immediate post-exercise period rather than during the exertion itself, it was found that levels of some adrenalins are much higher right after exercise. So one can assume that the same principle applies to the time period directly following a dangerous event.

- **Loss of status or self-esteem.** Deaths with loss of status or self-esteem included two men who were passed over for promotions they expected to get.

- **Emotional reunion or triumph.** Although it may not be surprising that a negatively charged event (like the threat of danger) can kill, it seems that too much of a good thing can be fatal as well: For instance, Engel included examples of death after reunions with loved ones, and the winning of a very large bet.

- **During mourning or on an anniversary of a death.** The examples Engel cited in this category included one of a man who dropped dead at the opening bars of a concert commemorating the death of his wife, a well-known piano teacher, five years earlier. The other was the case of a seventeen-year-old boy who died of a massive brain hemorrhage one year to the day, and within forty-eight minutes, of his older brother's untimely death in a car accident.

The age range of the people in Engel's examples spanned childhood through old age, but the majority were between fifty and eighty. The peak age of vulnerability was 45–55 for men, and 70–75 for women. Men were more likely to die in situations of danger; women's demises were more frequent after the loss of a loved one.

Engel also cites examples of animals dying under stress. A female llama died within minutes of seeing her mate of thirteen years shot and killed. Rats have been known to die of fright. Even cockroaches — despicable creatures though they may be — can be done in by being rendered helpless (by being pinned to a board) while facing danger in the form of a nearby, threatening dominant roach (ironically, also pinned down).

Engel references another author's work that included people who were convinced of the inevitability of their own deaths, "at a particular time or under particular circumstances, sometimes based on prediction made by fortune tellers years earlier." He feels that his data, although drawn from news reports, are reliable, as his cases are similar to others reported in the medical and lay literature. He believes that the common denominators are overwhelming excitation, loss of control, and giving up.

The paper concludes with speculation as to the physiology of death by emotion. Stress hormones, including adrenalin, speed the heart and make it electrically irritable so that potentially fatal rhythms may occur. Conversely, inhibition via other nerve pathways can slow the heart and may underlie the phenomenon of giving up or letting go. Engel feels that some interplay between sympathetic (excitatory) and parasympathetic (inhibitory) nervous systems, as well as higher, cerebral control mechanisms, must be involved. In 1971, when the work was published, it was not well known that spasms of the coronary arteries could occur. These can be reversible, and can also be sufficient to shut off blood flow to heart muscle so that a heart attack results. This was the presumed fate of the forty-year-old woman described in the *Lancet* nine years later, when the existence of these spasms was better known.

Oh, My Aching Heart

A recent article in the *New England Journal of Medicine* (February 10, 2005) took a hard, clinical look at the effects of sudden emotional stress on the heart. Nineteen patients (eighteen of them women) who developed cardiac symptoms such as chest pain, very difficult breathing, or cardiogenic shock right after emotional stress were evaluated. Their median age was sixty-three. The initiating event was often a family death, but one sixty-year-old woman was stricken because of a surprise party, in her honor. (I remember my uncle's terrified pallor on his 65th birthday when the lights went on and 165 guests shouted "surprise." He had a heart condition, and didn't look far from keeling over. Thankfully, he survived the shock and a good time was had by all.)

All of the nineteen patients in the article survived, and were studied in-hospital with coronary angiography (pictures of the heart-nourishing coronary arteries), echocardiography (an image of the heart made with sound waves), and, in some cases, blood levels of stress hormones like adrenalin; a few had biopsies of the heart muscle itself (known as myocardium). Only one of the patients actually had coronary artery disease —a predisposing condition. Adrenalin levels were much higher in these patients than in others admitted with actual heart attacks. The heart failed to pump adequately in all the patients, but this reversed in time. All these patients were still alive four years later. The authors call the condition "stress cardiomyopathy" or "myocardial stunning," but the exact mechanism remains unknown. Obviously the high adrenalin levels are involved, but we don't know precisely how.

A Will to Die

Besides deaths from sheer anxiety, Engel also is aware of Cannon's work, which I mentioned in the chapter on witchcraft, whereby someone appears to die by just letting go. In 1973, a *Lancet* article, "Self-Willed Death or the Bone-Pointing Syndrome," puts the experience of a physician at a melanoma clinic in Sydney, Australia into a wider perspective. Melanoma is a particularly nasty form of skin cancer. Often the prognosis is poor, and this clinic dealt with many patients who would not survive their disease. The writer, G. W. Milton, finds that "there is a small group of patients in whom the realization of impending death is a blow so terrible that they are quite unable to adjust to it, and they die rapidly before the malignancy seems to have developed enough to cause death." Milton describes this syndrome of self-willed death: A strong man, when first told of his malignancy, seems cavalier about it, but soon retreats. He loses interest in things, and while pulse, blood pressure, and respiration continue to be normal, he withdraws further and is dead within a month. Autopsy shows extensive cancer, but not sufficient to have killed the man at this time. Milton likens this to the bone-pointing voodoo deaths from the Australian outback, which I described in the witchcraft chapter (although these only took a few days for the patient to die).

Dr. Milton's depiction of self-willed death is very reminiscent of the patient, also in the witchcraft chapter, who seemed to be dying of cancer of the esophagus until his doctor convinced him, at least for the time being, that he was healthier than he realized. So . . . he walked out of the hospital. Milton's melanoma clinic sees patients who know that their cancer cannot be cured and are beginning to show signs of what he believes is self-willed death. And he notes that as soon as such a patient can be shown that something can be done to help, rapid improvement ensues.

The last angle from which the idea of self-willed death has been studied is statistical. It surprises me how many studies have been done that examined relationships, in retrospect, between when people die and when their birthdays are or which holidays were approaching or had passed; or relationships regarding other significant occasions. At least twenty publications address this, tabulating everything from birthdays to religious holidays to the harvest moon festival (older Chinese-American women were studied in that one). Many of the results are "positive," showing rises or dips before or after the symbolic event. But, like the studies on intercessory prayer, the data don't coincide very well. For instance, one examination of mortality relative to day of birth found death rates to be lower in females before the birthday and higher afterward; another paper reported the opposite. Male deaths, relative to birthdays, were also up/down in one survey, down/up in another.

A recent paper in the *Journal of the American Medical Association* (December 2004) looked at holidays, birthdays, and postponement of cancer deaths. The study looked at death certificates of 300,000 people in Ohio who had died of cancer over an eleven-year period. No evidence was found that cancer patients postponed their deaths to see just one more big day, as previous studies had suggested.

So where does this leave us with regard to the banker, the Spartan, and the mother of five whose stories I presented in detail? The forty-year-old mother managed to actually have a heart attack, unlike the suddenly frightened, myocardially "stunned" women who, like her, had normal coronary arteries. She timed her exit perfectly, just as she had predicted three days in advance. This doesn't quite fit the syndrome of self-willed withdrawal or that of the hyperexcited collapse. But somehow, she knew. The bank vice-president, the Greek immigrant—they knew (God knows how). And without a single sign of deterioration, anxiety, shock, or awe, they departed this world at precisely the right second, as if Struck Down.

ℕine

Moving Toward the Light:
Near-Death Experiences

Raymond Moody had a Ph.D. in philosophy and then went on to become a medical doctor and psychiatrist. His 1975 book *Life After Life* first used the term "near-death experience" (NDE) to describe a phenomenon sometimes seen in people who have almost, but not quite, died. Such experiences, typically described as going toward a bright light or coursing through a tunnel, are part of folklore, and have been depicted historically and across cultures. Swiss geologist Albert von St. Gallen Heim, an avid mountain climber, had some sort of "experience" after a bad fall in 1871. This prompted him to speak to other climbers, and in 1892 he published *Notes on Deaths from Falls* which contains accounts of nearly-fatal accidents that were somehow survived amid visions of enlightenment.

"Near-death experience" must have been a good fit for the examples in Heim's anthology, because this term stuck. NDEs have been the subject of much study, and while their meaning is controversial, the number of people who believe they have had them makes it possible for statistics and data to be collected.

A Wakening in the O.R.

Let's begin with a well-documented and detailed account, written by Georgia cardiologist Dr. Michael Sabom in his 1998 book *Light and Death: One Doctor's Fascinating Account of Near-Death Experiences.*[3] Sabom was rather skeptical at first about NDEs but, after many patient interviews, changed his mind. This patient was a thirty-five-year-old woman who was found to have a large aneurysm (a balloon-like swelling) in her brain; if it ruptured—a real possibility—she would almost certainly die. An "extraordinary" neurosurgical procedure was her only hope. This would involve diverting all blood away from her brain for about forty-five minutes, allowing the surgeons to make the repair. Since a brain cannot live without oxygen-supplying blood for more than a few minutes, something rather special had to be done. First, her body temperature had to be lowered to 60 degrees Fahrenheit, which isn't all that chilly if you're outside on a sunny spring day while you maintain the temperature inside the body at the usual 98.6 degrees—but this woman's *body* temperature was going to be 60 degrees. That freezes all bodily functions and all cellular activity, including brain cells.

This was accomplished by a cardiopulmonary bypass machine, a mechanical heart and lung through which all the patient's blood was diverted. The blood was tapped from a large artery in the groin (the femoral artery) into the machine, where

3 Grand Rapids, MI: Zondervan, pp. 37–51, 1998.

it was cooled to 60 degrees and then returned to the body through a vein. Ultimately, the body's "core" temperature became 60 degrees. Then all blood was drained from her head, collapsing the aneurysm so that it could be fixed without the bother of having blood rushing through. During this time, the patient was "clinically dead"; there was zero brain electrical activity (the EEG was a flat line), and her heart had stopped. Even the lowest centers of her brain (known as the brain stem) had ceased function. The only difference between this and really being dead is that this state was induced and reversible.

The significance of this in the context of a discussion of near-death experience is that her physiologic state was carefully monitored, documenting known parameters of lifelessness. Many NDE reports lack this, allowing the possibility that the person wasn't as close to dying as it may have seemed. But this woman was clearly in a state in which she could not hear (the brain wouldn't respond), nor could she have had seizure activity (her EEG, which would register this if it happened, was flat). Whatever she perceived could not have come through the senses, or from nerve or cell activity, as there was none.

Here is what this clinically dead woman reported: The noise of the saw used to cut through her skull awakened her from the anesthesia. She felt herself pulled out of her body through the hole in her head, and could watch the proceedings from a vantage point above the neurosurgeon's shoulder. She supplied details about the pneumatic saw used for cutting, and knew of a problem the cardiac surgeon had had in finding an appropriate vessel for the shunting procedure. She knew what music was being played in the operating room. At the juncture when her heart stopped, she passed through a tunnel toward a brilliant light. There she met several deceased relatives who advised her to go back, lest she not survive the surgery.

NDE Analysis

Enough people have recounted stories like this so that common features can be tabulated for comparison. Remembrances are similar but not identical. Moody originally listed fifteen elements of NDEs, including seeing a dark tunnel, feeling out of one's body, meeting spiritual beings, experiencing a bright light, and a sense of returning to the body.

Dr. Moody began his residency training in psychiatry at the University of Virginia during the 1970s, just as his book became popular. He promptly received enough letters from readers who had had NDEs to fill a box, and he showed these to a junior faculty member, Bruce Greyson, who then became interested in the phenomenon.

Dr. Greyson, currently a professor of psychiatry at UVA, published a "near-death experience scale" in a 1983 paper in the *Journal of Nervous and Mental Disease.* Previous observers like Moody had listed what seemed like consistent, crucial elements of NDEs, but Greyson wanted a scientific tool that could be easily administered by clinicians.

So he took sixty-seven subjects who claimed to have had NDEs and gave them an eighty-item questionnaire. Responses were then culled down to sixteen items felt to be the most clinically meaningful. These final sixteen questions were those most often answered affirmatively, and where responses were consistent when the test was given a second time a few months later. The questionnaire consisted of four headings with four questions within each category:

Cognitive

- Did time seem to speed up?

- Were your thoughts speeded up?

- Did scenes from your past come back to you?

- Did you suddenly seem to understand everything?

Affective

- Did you have a feeling of peace and pleasantness?

- Did you have a feeling of joy?

- Did you feel a sense of unity or harmony with the universe?

- Did you see, or feel surrounded by, a brilliant light?

Paranormal

- Were your senses more vivid than usual?

- Did you seem to be aware of things going on elsewhere (ESP)?

- Did scenes from the future come to you?

- Did you feel separated from your physical body?

Transcendental

- Did you seem to enter some other, unearthly world?

- Did you seem to encounter a mystical being or presence?

- Did you see deceased spirits or religious figures?

- Did you come to a border or point of no return?

Answers were weighted 0, 1, or 2, depending on degree of concurrence. A score of 7 or more was considered significant for research purposes. The subject's age, sex, and amount of time elapsed since the NDE event had no effect on responses. Of note, the passage through a tunnel, frequently an NDE component, was not used, as Greyson found that it did not correlate well with the other parameters. He did feel that this final sixteen-piece scale was reliable and could differentiate true NDEs from brain damage or diseases and from stress reactions following recovery from a dangerous situation.

Two years later, Greyson published a "typology" of NDEs. Having developed a scale that simply identified an event as an NDE, he now wanted to see if there were differing NDE types. Greyson analyzed eighty-nine claimed NDEs, using his sixteen-part instrument as described above, and was able to "cluster" the responses into three types. Forty-three percent scored highest on the transcendental component, 42 percent emerged as affective, and the remaining 15 percent were predominantly cognitive. Neither age nor gender seemed to make a difference, nor did the medical specifics of the near-death event itself. What did seem to matter was whether the "death" was sudden and unexpected (accident, cardiac arrest), or anticipated (terminal illness, surgery). Cognitive features, like seeing one's entire life in a flash, seemed to accompany the former, but were lacking from the latter, as if death's slower approach had already allowed time for life-review.

Michael Sabom, the cardiologist who reported the aneurysm case, reviewed a series of NDEs and categorized them as "autoscopic," meaning a sense of looking down at oneself from above, and transcendental (see above). About a third were autoscopic, slightly more than half were transcendental, and the rest had features of both.

NDEs in the Not-Near-Dead

What happens if someone thinks they are close to death, but they really aren't? This was the question posed by Ph.D. psychologist Justine Owens and colleagues at the University of Virginia in their 1990 publication in *Lancet*. "Features of NDE in Relation to Whether or Not Patients Were Near Death" examined the medical records of fifty-eight patients, twenty-eight of whom were judged to have been so close to death that they would have died without medical intervention. The other thirty were not in danger of dying, although they believed they were.

What were the differences? Seventy-five percent of the truly near-death patients experienced a bright light; forty percent of those not actually near death did as well. These differences are significant, statistically speaking. Also significant (i.e., unlikely to have occurred by chance) was enhanced cognitive function in the nearly-dead group. Not measurably different were the tunnel experience, a sense of having exited the body and viewing it from above, and life-review. The authors note that the enhancement of thought processes (cognitive function) was greater in the people really near-death, who would have had diminished brain function. Those who only thought they were having a close brush, who would have had normal brain function, were less likely to have had clear, comprehensive thinking.

Merely fainting can occasionally cause NDE features. A 1994 letter to *Lancet* described a study where syncope (a doctors' term for fainting) was induced in forty-two healthy young adults by having them hyperventilate and then pushing to exhale with the mouth tightly closed (we call this a Valsalva maneuver). This briefly cuts off blood flow and, consequently, oxygen to the brain and causes one to faint. When I was a teenager in the late 1950s, we didn't have drugs, so we occasionally amused ourselves by fainting, using the same method. The *Lancet* volunteers frequently reported visual and auditory hallucinations and an occasional out-of-body experience. Most described the overall feeling as pleasurable. When we did it, there was something vaguely pleasant about the experience, although no one ever said anything about odd perceptions; as an amusement, it got old fast.

The Real McCoy

Australian sociologist Allan Kellehear studied NDEs in non-Western societies, particularly India and China, to look for common elements across cultures. The tunnel experience was not found. Unifying features included a sense of other beings or of another world. Combining Kellehear's data with Owens's and the syncope report, one gets a sense of core aspects of what human beings undergo, sometimes, when truly near death: a bright light, clarity of thinking, and another world.

Polls and Probabilities

So, how many people have had NDEs, and what is your likelihood, if resuscitated, of reporting one? A Gallup poll, published in 1982, found 5 percent of the adult American population to have had such an experience, which they said represented about half those resuscitated. I find these figures a little difficult to accept, not so much because no one I know has ever told me they've had one, but because it would mean that 10 percent of the adult population in 1982 had at some point teetered on the very edge of life. A *U.S. News & World Report* poll in the March 31, 1997, issue claims that eighteen percent of Americans believed that they had once been on the verge of dying. I again find this high, to say the least. Greyson's sixteen-point scale wasn't used for these surveys, allowing for the possibility that many of the reported experiences would not have qualified as research-grade NDEs. As we saw in the *Lancet* paper above, people often describe near-death phenomena when in fact, they only *thought* they had cheated the grim reaper.

There is more recent, scientifically rigorous work on the subject. Dr. Sam Parnia, a physician and university researcher at Southampton General Hospital in England, along with his colleagues, surveyed all survivors of cardiac arrest at their hospital during an entire year. This 2001 study was prospective, meaning planned in advance, which is generally considered more valid than retrospective, where you go back and look afterward. The surviving patients were interviewed within a week of the arrest. Of sixty-three such patients, seven (11 percent) reported memories, four with NDE features.

Another prospective study, published the same year in *Lancet*, came from the Netherlands, where 344 consecutive patients at ten Dutch hospitals who had been successfully revived were interviewed within a few days of suffering cardiac arrest. A previously published scoring system was used, although not Greyson's. These patients had been clinically dead, defined as "a period of unconsciousness caused by insufficient oxygen supply to the brain." After a few minutes of oxygen deprivation, irreparable brain damage occurs. Of the 344 subjects studied, sixty-two (18 percent) had some remembrance at the time of clinical death. Since none of the 344 patients was getting oxygen to his/her brain during the arrests, the authors (cardiologist Pim van Lommel and colleagues) felt that dire medical straits alone could not account for these remembrances, since the majority of the people studied had neither NDEs nor any recollections around the cardiac arrest.

When the patients' memories were scored, two-thirds of the recollections qualified as NDEs, which means that twelve percent overall had them. These twelve percent were no sicker than, nor medically distinguishable from, the others. Dr. van Lommel wonders if society's negative attitude toward NDEs could deter people from reporting them, making their incidence appear lower. He concludes, at any rate, that "we do not know why so few patients report NDE" after resuscitation, and that a "purely physiological explanation" (such as lack of brain oxygen or activity) fails to correlate with who will have them.

Bruce Greyson published a 2003 paper about a survey done in a cardiac inpatient unit at a Virginia hospital. Over thirty months, all those admitted to the cardiac care unit—almost sixteen hundred in all—were evaluated for NDEs. Seven percent of these admissions suffered cardiac arrest, and one out of ten of these described an NDE. By contrast, one out of a hundred cardiac patients who did not have an arrest reported one.

Greyson has more recently estimated the percentage of

Americans who will report an NDE after being truly near death to be between 9 and 18 percent. Obviously, it matters whether or not the person really was near, or if the memories meet NDE criteria. Most of the studies seem to come up with similar numbers. I can't say that any of my own patients ever volunteered any sort of NDE to me. Then again, my practice is largely outpatient, so I'm not usually dealing with the critically ill; and, as mentioned above, this is not something that's ordinarily talked about by patients or physicians.

When Dr. Jeffrey P. Long emailed over five hundred physicians at Brown University Medical Center to inquire about their views on patients' NDEs, only 3 percent bothered to respond. In 1977, when Michael Sabom was at the University of Florida College of Medicine in Gainesville, he reported on eleven patients with NDE descriptions consistent with what had been published elsewhere. At the same time, he also took an informal survey of the medical center physicians, who seemed to have no awareness of such events in gravely ill patients. In a 1980 letter of reply to Dr. Sabom in *JAMA*, physician Richard Blacher of the Tufts University School of Medicine stated that he had interviewed several thousand patients who had undergone cardiac and heart surgery without ever having had such an episode described. I don't know if each beholder's eye saw things differently, or if the way the questions were asked influenced the response. A lot goes on under our noses, medically speaking, that our patients don't tell us about.

The Non-Association of Mind and Body

What sort of a person is likely to report an NDE, given the appropriate circumstances? In Greyson's chapter on NDEs in a 2000 publication by the American Psychological Association,[4] he comments that few personal traits have been identified that can predict who will have an NDE or which type they will have. Experiencers tend to be psychologically healthy and no different from non-experiencers in age, sex, race, or religion. Dr. Greyson wrote a *Lancet* paper the same year asking the question: "Dissociation in people who have near-death experiences: out of their bodies or out of their minds?" As I mentioned in chapter 7 on possession, there is a psychiatric classification known as dissociative disorders, meaning the patient displays a dissociation (i.e., separation) between what's going on in the mind and what's actually happening. Daydreaming is a non-pathological form of dissociation. Pathological dissociation includes trances, stress-induced amnesia, and multiple personality disorder, things where the patient's "reality" is so separated from normal consciousness and memory as to appear quite unreal to anyone else. Obviously, an NDE, which involves floating above and away from bleak reality, would qualify.

Greyson employed a commonly used psychiatric screening instrument for dissociation, the dissociative experiences scale (DES), and sent it to ninety-six people who had reported an NDE, and to an additional thirty-eight who had come close to death but had no NDE (these thirty-eight would be a comparison, or control, group). The DES is a twenty-eight-item scale that grades intensity of dissociative-type experiences, and scores of thirty or higher usually indicate a dissociative disorder. In this study, the NDE patients had a median score of 10.7; the non-NDE sample's median was 7.3. Although these are significantly different, both are well below the pathological cutoff.

4 In: *Varieties of Anomalous Experience 2000.* American Psychological Association, Washington, D.C.

Greyson concludes that NDEs are not pathological and not part of a dissociative disorder, and that they are a normal stress response that some people undergo—in other words, "out of their bodies," not minds.

The Aftermath

Okay, you've returned from the brink and you remember a divine, albeit bizarre, scenario. What is life like from here on in? This is the part that surprised me from researching NDEs: A lot of people seemed to be better off. This was not invariably true, but several observers have noted a positive change. In the Netherlands study of 344 resuscitated patients (which had compared NDE-ers with the merely uncon-scious), experiencers were more likely to come out with an increased belief in an afterlife and a lessened fear of death— which may not be surprising, considering what they went through. They were also found at follow-up to have "gone through a positive change, and were more self-assured, socially aware, and religious than before." Greyson, in a 1993 publication in the journal *Psychiatry,* comments about the "long-lasting changes in values, beliefs, and behavior" that have been seen.

Some studies suggest that it may take a while until what seems to have happened fully sinks in. How a patient's family, friends, and physicians react can make the difference between having had a transforming experience versus a brief immersion in psy-chosis. Sabom, in his original eleven-case review, writes that such a patient "is often relieved at being able to discuss his expe-rience in an atmosphere of openness and understanding and is comforted with the knowledge that others have had similar encounters." Unfortunately, you can't always count on finding an attitude of openness and understanding; so reveal that near-death epiphany at your own risk. I was hesitant to even ask a patient (the one time I tried) about a possible NDE; if I had had one myself, I'd hesitate even more. Fortunately, I'm not aware that I've ever been near death (I'm not counting that creepy feeling you get before general anesthesia), but I suppose if I had opened death's door, looked inside, and gone back home, I'd be a changed and more spiritual fellow.

Biologic Explanations

Biologic explanations as to why NDEs might occur are reviewed by Greyson in his book chapter, mentioned above. Many of the references are in the *Journal of Near-Death Studies*, which is not MEDLINE-indexed but contains scientific work. Are NDE's figments of one's imagination? Greyson believes that people who have never heard or read about NDEs, including children, have nevertheless described them, with typical features. Does the NDE simply reflect the brain's reaction to lack of oxygen? Sabom's aneurysm patient had, temporarily, a dead brain, devoid of *any* ability to react. And most patients with oxygen-deprived brains do not have NDEs. Brain chemistry gone awry is another hypothesis. Endorphins — naturally occurring brain opiates — have been postulated to cause NDEs; but giving patients opiates, such as morphine, does not induce true NDE features. Michael Persinger, a Canadian neurobiologist mentioned in other places in this book, can induce many aspects of an NDE by applying external electric or magnetic fields to the head of an awake person, although the totality of an NDE does not occur. (A Swedish team, however, was unable to replicate Persinger's findings.) In fact, Greyson concludes that "No theory had yet been proposed that can account satisfactorily for all the common elements of NDEs."

British lecturer and psychologist Susan Blackmore is a fellow of the United Kingdom skeptics' organization and has also been an officer of the Society for Psychical Research. In her 1996 paper in the *Journal of the Royal Society of Medicine,* she examines six extant medical or psychological theories of NDEs, finds them all inadequate, and remarks that while there's no evidence that NDEs indicate a reality of survival after death, the experiences can't be dismissed as fantasy or as a by-product of medical intervention.

NDEs in Children

And then there are the children. Much of this work has been done by Seattle pediatrician Melvin Morse. In 1983, he reported a near-death experience, with the usual trimmings, in a seven-year-old child who had almost drowned. Three years later, in the same *American Journal of Diseases of Children,* he wrote up a series of eleven children, aged three through sixteen, who had survived life-threatening illness; seven had memories of the NDE type. An additional twenty-nine children, matched for age, were sick enough to be in an intensive-care unit and unconscious, but were not deemed close to dying. None of this group had any recollection of the time they were unconscious. Morse also makes note of the differences between adult and pediatric NDEs. Children were less likely to have time distortions or to undergo a life-review. While adults tended to meet dead relatives and friends, children reported meeting living teachers and friends. Children's parents, for some reason, seemed never to appear in their

NDEs. Like adults, Morse believes children survive an NDE with a new, more serene life outlook.

So what does this all mean? How does someone emerge from general anesthesia and a brain-dead coma and accurately describe concurrent operating-room events? Why do some doctors encounter patients with NDEs with relative frequency, while others never see or hear of such a patient? Is it just a question of being receptive? Why can some people experience NDE features without actually being near death, or by merely fainting, or by just having their brain stimulated by a magnetic field? When these answers are known, the "near-death experience" will no longer be paranormal.

$\mathcal{T}$en

I Remember It Well: The Collective Unconscious and the Nature of Memory

Logic tells us that what each human being "knows" comes from individual learning and life experience. But are there experiences and memories that all human beings—no matter what race, creed, or country of origin—share? In 1906, thirty-one-year-old Swiss psychiatrist Carl Gustav Jung (who would ultimately become world-famous for his theories of psychotherapy and personality, founding the field of analytic psychology and coining the terms "introvert" and "extrovert") encountered what he considered a "curious delusion"[5] while examining a schizophrenic patient residing in a mental hospital.

5 Jung, C. G. *The Collected works of C.G. Jung.* In: *The Archetypes and the Collective Unconscious;* vol. 9. Princeton: Princeton University Press, 1959:50–52.

The Vision

The patient was a man in his thirties who suffered from a paranoid form of psychosis that had begun in his early twenties. Before being institutionalized, he had been an ordinary man who worked as an office clerk. During active periods of illness, he suffered from hallucinations or became megalomaniacal and thought himself to be the Savior. In quieter times, he was allowed to roam the corridors of the institution, which is where Dr. Jung encountered him at a window one day, staring at the sun and moving his head oddly to and fro.

The patient called the doctor over to the window and asked him to look at the sun, through half-closed eyes, in order to appreciate the "sun's penis"—the horizontal, almost tubular yellow glow as it would appear through the squint. Then he had the doctor turn his head from side to side, to make the "penis" move, and claimed this movement to be the origin of the wind.

Jung found no particular meaning in this madman's vision; but, like any good scientist, he made note of it. Four years later, Jung was studying mythology when he read about a recently translated ancient Greek papyrus in which an essentially identical vision was described. In the Greek text, a tube from which the wind is created hangs down from the sun, a windstream emanating from it. The author even intends for the reader to experience this illusion as it appears "through the disc of the sun."

The Collective Unconscious: The Thoughts We All Share

Although the first printing of the Greek translation was in 1903, this patient had been committed well before then and could not possibly have seen it. He had never traveled and was not highly educated. How did an institutionalized man come up with this?

Jung postulated a "collective unconscious": a universal human consciousness that holds the collective memories, experiences, and wisdom of the human race, and into which certain people are able to tap. This would be distinct from the personal unconscious, assembled from memories of this lifetime. To Jung, this primordial memory bank explained how vastly different cultures living in different eras could construct myths and fables — of heroes and villains, of struggles between good and evil — that were otherwise inexplicably similar to each other.

In addition to the "sun's penis" example, Jung related the story of a girl who stated that she had a black snake in her belly. To Jung, this was a symbol from the collective unconscious, as the concept of a serpent within the body existed in India (unknown to this girl) as Kundalini — a latent, coiled energy at the base of the spine. Even ideas of power, God, spirit, and the soul were seen as universal and innate within all of homo sapiens and throughout history, not as things learned during any one individual's lifetime.

Jung also believed that the emergence of the concept of conservation of energy had somehow percolated up from the collective unconscious. Nowadays, energy conservation (also called the first law of thermodynamics) is elementary physics. But this principle — that energy is neither created nor destroyed, but only changes form — had eluded Galileo and Newton and was not fully accepted until the end of the nineteenth century. What's more, it was simultaneously and independently discovered during the first half of that century by at least six individuals, none of whom were physicists, and all of whom met with much resistance. One of the six, physician Robert Mayer, is generally credited with the idea. Jung cites an 1844 letter of Mayer's regarding the genesis of this theorem. Mayer was a ship's doctor in the tropics who preferred to stay on board rather than go exploring. Here he could reflect peacefully, and describes "flashes of thought" that "came to the surface." These inspirations culminated in Mayer's epiphany. To Jung, "the idea of energy and its conservation must be a primordial image that was dormant in the collective unconscious."[6]

Freud also believed in "a collective mind, in which mental processes occur just as they do in the mind of an individual. In particular, I have supposed that the sense of guilt for an action has persisted for many thousands of years and has remained operative in generations which can have had no knowledge of that action."[7]

What's the status of the collective unconscious these days? A March 2005 search of the MEDLINE database, using the phrase "collective unconscious" as the search term, turned up twenty-three results published between 1984 and 2004. Here are a few of the most interesting:

- In a 1984 article from a German psychiatric journal, the author relates the case of an adolescent in the throes of severe depression, whose drawings, sandplays, and dreams are compared by the author to the symbols used in primitives' initiation rites. "Astonishing parallels are found," in terms of the basic motifs, which the author feels are manifestations of the collective unconscious.

- From the *Journal of Analytic Psychology*, we have "Primordial Image and the Archetypal Design of Art," in which the writer notes that while lower primates can draw, only humans create pictorial representations—i.e., images of things that really exist. Jung's work refers

6 Storr, A. In: *The Essential Jung*. New York: MJF Books, 1983: 68–69.

7 Freud S. Standard, ed. *An Outline of Psychoanalysis*; vol. XIII. London: The Hogarth Press, 1964: 157–158.

to primordial images (archetypes) peculiar to our entire species, spontaneously generated, and consistent throughout time and geographic area. Often these archetypes contain dual and opposing images—the wise old man and the youth; the hermaphrodite. The author of this article analyzes double-figure art imagery from prehistoric and modern societies, which potentially validate Jung's postulates.

• In a slightly different vein is "Antisemitism and Jung's Concept of the Collective Unconscious," a letter from two Austrian doctors to the *American Journal of Psychiatry,* noting that the mechanism of transmission of Jung's archetypes, over many generations, "excludes rigorous experimental analysis." They feel that the pervasiveness, particularly over time, of anti-Semitism may qualify it as a Jungian entity.

• "The Perspective of the Female Archetype in Nursing" comes from Portugal, where two researchers feel that this profession has not changed much throughout its history. They believe that the essence of nursing—caring—is a feminine archetype from the collective unconscious, associated with the protection, promotion, and preservation of the human being. I must say that while over half the entrants to American medical schools these days are women (versus ten percent when I entered school thirty-five years ago), the nursing profession still remains overwhelmingly female.

• Lastly, in an article describing the healing rituals of the Xhosa-speaking peoples of South Africa, reverence of ancestors is stressed, body and mind are linked through dancing and drumming, and the community participates. The author believes the ancestors to be archetypal representations of the collective unconscious.

Despite the fact that the collective unconscious may still be a part of modern psychiatric philosophy, a system where memories and images spring from a communal repository—rather than from direct experiences during one's actual lifetime — did not slide smoothly down the gullets of the scientific cognoscenti. Jung was much criticized for his collective unconscious because of what it implied: that people "knew" or "remembered" things that they hadn't learned or experienced. Were these concepts encoded into our DNA, like animals' instincts? Could they enter the brain (i.e., consciousness) from without, like a far-away broadcast enters your radio, if properly tuned, through its antenna? What is, in fact, the nature of memory, and where is it stored?

I Remember it Well

Believe it or not, we don't quite know how memories are kept in the brain. They are not site-specific, like on your hard drive, and this has been frustrating for neuroscientists. While certain anatomic areas of the brain are involved in processing and storage of memories, no area can be found that stores a specific memory. Shepherd Franz, an American neuropsychologist who experimented with cats and monkeys and with humans with brain lesions, concluded in 1912 that the exact localization of mental processes in the brain is impossible.

Franz's student Karl Lashley taught rats to find their way through a maze (for food, of course), and then damaged different parts of their cerebral cortex (where the higher brain functions reside) to see which parts might be responsible for the maze-memories. Lashley found that the *amount* of tissue damaged, rather than its location, impacted the rats' retention. He concluded, in 1929, that all cortical areas were equipotential (equal) for learning, and could substitute for each other where learning was concerned; he also found the reduction in learning to be proportional to the amount of tissue destroyed. In other words, the more cortex obliterated, the longer it took the rat to find the food, regardless of where the damage occurred. Lashley felt, ironically, that the only legitimate scientific conclusion, after thirty years of research, was that memory was theoretically impossible, since it could not be localized.

Lashley's work is reminiscent of the hologram, long into the future, where the entire picture can be regenerated from any of its parts, the only caveat being: the smaller the part, the less clear the picture.

I am always amazed by the amount of human brain that can be removed without removing any specific memories. A physician colleague of mine suffered from temporal lobe epilepsy, and medication failed to control his seizures, as is sometimes the case with this type of epilepsy. In this situation, as a last resort, brain surgery can be performed, to remove the tissue from which the electrical chaos emanates: the epileptic focus (which we usually *can* localize). Two inches of my colleague's right temporal lobe was excised. Although this is a brain area intimately involved with memory, not only didn't my colleague lose any memories, but he actually felt that his memory got better after the surgery, as he no longer needed to take anti-epileptic medications that fogged his recall.

The Brain, the Mind, and the Neurosurgeon

The Canadian neurosurgeon Wilder Penfield pioneered this type of surgery. Beginning in the late 1930s, he was able to stimulate the brain's surface directly, with a weak electrical current, to find the seizure focus. Since the brain contains no pain sensors, the skull can be entered using local anesthesia, meaning Penfield's patients could remain awake while this was done. (Nowadays, high-resolution MRI scans and other closed-skull techniques localize the seizure focus; my colleague had general anesthesia.)

Penfield knew that in the throes of a temporal lobe–based seizure, visual or auditory hallucinations sometimes occur, and this rendered him even more curious as to what effect localized electrical stimulation of various parts of the brain would produce. Since his patients were able to converse during the surgery, Penfield had only to ask them what they experienced. It turned out that the reaction of subjects to focal brain stimulation was generally unpredictable. Repeated stimulation of the same spot evoked responses of the same sensory modality (e.g., visual or auditory), but the content generally differed. Sometimes you could stimulate the same spot on the brain any number of times and get a different reaction in every instance. For example, in a 1963 report on the surgery of a twenty-one-year-old man, several stimuli of a single point in the temporal lobe produced the following reactions, respectively:

"Like footsteps walking, on the radio."

"Like company in the room."

". . . like being in a dance hall . . . at the gymnasium—like at Kenwood High School."

". . . like a lady was talking to a child."

"Radio. I think it was Philadelphia; it was news."

It was as if this man's "radio," tuned to the same channel, was picking up different stations every time it was turned on.

Penfield noticed some other interesting things about direct brain stimulation. Within the temporal lobes, it produced "interpretive illusions," like those of the patient above. These often were auditory, and they seemed to evoke memory snippets from the patient's past. (In some cases, it could not be proved that the experiences were actually from the patient's past, although usually they were.) But excitation in other brain areas, like those for speech or vision, did not produce words or images from the past, and Penfield could find no area of the brain where his activation could cause a patient to believe or to decide. This was judgment, the province of the mind.

His 1975 book *The Mystery of the Mind* was published shortly before he died. Penfield had become fascinated by the fact that his electrical probes could not, in essence, locate a person's mind. He believed it was "impossible to explain the mind on the basis of neuronal action within the brain" and that "a second fundamental element and a second form of energy" must exist.

Magnetic Fields and Memory

Electrical stimulation is not the only tool scientists have used to try to unlock the mysteries of memory. Michael A. Persinger, the neurophysiologist in Ontario, Canada, employed an external device (which has obvious practical advantages over poking into the naked brain) to examine memory processing. Subjects listened to a short narrative during which they were exposed to weak, non-perceptible low-frequency magnetic fields from a device applied externally to the side of the head. Direct recall was unaffected, but the number of inferences made from the story doubled in the exposed group, compared with sham-treated controls, suggesting an influence on the details of recall. Persinger's work on magnetic fields and memory will be the subject of a later chapter.

Finally, in "Are Neuronal Activity–Associated Magnetic Fields the Physical Base for Memory?" (*Medical Hypotheses,*

2002), M. A. M. Banaclocha, from the pathology department in Castellon, Spain, speculates that information could be stored in the brain in the form of magnetic fields, similar to the way videotape holds data. Normal brain activity produces measurable electricity, which in turn produces weak electromagnetic fields (EMF's); there is abundant evidence that externally applied, weak EMF's affect cellular function. And there is a line of research that found magnetite—the naturally occurring iron-based mineral of which the first magnets were composed—to be widely distributed in human brains, so magnetic storage is plausible. (Scientists at the California Institute of Technology first documented magnetite in human brain tissue in 1992. Previously it had been known to exist in bacteria and lower animals.)

We do know that there are different types of memory. Recalling what you had for breakfast this morning, the names of your children, and how to drive a car all depend on different areas of the brain and are affected by different diseases. A patient of mine—a man in his mid-seventies, with Alzheimer's disease so severe that he could not remember, ten seconds afterward, that I had given him a flu shot—drove a car with no problems, as long as his wife, sitting beside him, fed him the directions (I don't recommend this). We know that certain parts of the brain are more intimately involved than others in our abilities to store and retrieve memories (we just don't know quite where the vault might be). The temporal lobes, on the sides of the cortex, where Penfield performed his stimulations, are needed for normal recall, as are the hippocampi (seahorse-shaped structures) beneath them. Injuries to both hippocampi destroy short-term memory, the fate of the main character in the movie *Memento* (Columbia Tri-Star, 2000). Interestingly, magnetic material has been found in the hippocampi, and even visualized there through sophisticated microscopy.

So, while we in the twenty-first century know a lot more about brain function and anatomy than Jung knew at the turn of the twentieth, we still don't know enough about the physiology of memory to prove or refute his theory of memory collectively shared by all of humankind.

$\mathcal{E}$leven

Partying with the Devil: Satanic Ritual Abuse

Where, exactly, do memories go? You have an experience, you learn something; where is this knowledge stored? In the brain, we presume, but don't try to locate the memory in any particular spot: you can't. Only the brain's apparatus for storing and retrieving information is anatomically understood.

And where, exactly, do memories come from? The obvious answer is from life experiences; but, like Jung's collective unconscious, there are many remembrances that just don't seem to jive with things past.

Remembering Satan

Consider the tragic case of the Ingram family of Olympia, Washington, beginning in 1988, as written by Lawrence Wright in *The New Yorker* ("Remembering Satan," May 1993).

Paul Ingram, forty-three, was a family man, a religious man, and a model citizen. Then two of his daughters (he had five children) accused him of repeated sexual abuse. That's the "normal" part of the story; the rest just gets weirder.

The allegations began when the older daughter Ericka, twenty-two, attended a two-day fundamentalist church retreat led by a charismatic Christian "healer," during which memories of childhood sexual abuse by her father were evoked. There are some differences between the police report and eyewitness accounts of what happened at the retreat, but Wright's narrative describes a "mesmerized" group of sixty girls, two of whom suddenly recalled childhood sexual abuse before Ericka's revelations emerged. The actual evocation process consisted of the healer, believing that she (the healer) was being prompted by the Lord, telling Ericka that she (Ericka) had been sexually abused as a child. In Wright's account, taken from the healer, Ericka never spoke.

Thus began a chain of events that spread like an out-of-control fire. A few months later, Ericka told her mother of repeated sexual molestation by her father, and now included the victimization of two of her brothers as well. Her sister Julie, eighteen, told of suffering the same sort of abuse. The police interviewed both girls, then arrested their father. Although he could not remember ever sexually abusing any of his children, Paul Ingram believed that if his daughters accused him of this, it must be true. In essence, he confessed to crimes he did not remember committing.

With prodding from his interrogators, Paul recovered dream-like scenarios of having sex with his daughters, specifying what he "would've" done rather than what he *had* done. The events unfolded to him, in his words, "like I'm watching a movie." He assumed that he had repressed what he had done, and that "there may be a dark side of me that I don't know about." Throughout these proceedings, he remained emotionless and detached, in a way quite unlike any that the police had seen before in this type of crime.

The dark side got darker. Ingram believed he housed a demon and asked his pastor for an exorcism (some mild modification, aimed at evicting bad spirits, was arranged). Then he had memories of people in robes kneeling around a fire, perhaps with the Devil on hand. The daughters had never mentioned satanic rituals in their accusations. (That would change.) Meanwhile, they implicated two of their father's friends, frequently at the house for poker games. Ingram, under questioning, was able to provide recovered details of sex acts with his daughters that also involved these friends. One of the men, confronted, remembered nothing of the sort, but allowed for the possibility that he could have unconsciously obliterated such horror from his brain.

Paul's wife also did not believe the allegations made by her daughters. But then she too came to doubt the reliability of her own memory. In some of Ericka's accounts, her mother had even been an observer of, and participant in, the abuse. What a thing not to remember!

The oldest son Chad, twenty, was then located (he had left home a few years earlier and was estranged from the family). He expressed dislike for his father but did not recall any sexual abuse within the household, nor any recollection of having been abused himself, despite his father's claim that Chad, too, had been a victim. Questioned by police, "a now familiar fixated expression came over his [Chad's] face," according to Wright, and "his voice took on the monotonous quality of a trance-like state." (Police notes also mention a "trance-like state.") Under suggestion that something horrible had happened to him that was repressed within his memory, the memories came. Repeated sexual abuse, often by some kind of cult, had occurred during most of his life. The father's two poker buddies were also involved: Chad remembered seeing his mother tied spread-eagle to a bed, having sex acts performed by her husband and his friends.

Enter Satan. About a month after Ingram's arrest, Ericka wrote out a detailed statement describing a satanic ritual involving many people, including her parents. Part of this ritual, among other things, was the sacrifice of a live human baby. Ingram had alluded to the possibility of an evil within, but now came the gory details. Ericka described sexual acts with goats and dogs, repeatedly from kindergarten to high school, in which her mother was sometimes included. She described orgies in the woods in which babies were sacrificed and buried, and estimated that she had attended eight hundred and fifty rituals and had watched the sacrifices of no less than twenty-five babies.

Many of the abuse particulars involved cuts and incisions on the two daughters, at least some of which would be expected to leave scars. These were, in fact, looked for, but never found. Human sacrifices leave behind blood and bodies. The Ingram property was dug up in a search for just such traces. None were found, even though the girls had provided maps of where to look. The details of each family member's accounts of the abuse never coincided, with discrepancies of dates, persons present, and events. Ericka herself was not consistent in her stories. Two academic psychologists were called in to evaluate the situation, and their determination was that the abuse had never happened.

But Paul Ingram was convicted and did his time: fourteen years in prison. There are some who believe that satanic cults are commonly operative in the United States, and the Ingram case is just one example. Ingram's prosecutors believe he was justly convicted. He, however, no longer believes he had any involvement in sexual abuse of his children, ritualistic or otherwise. His younger daughter, Julie, has recanted, at least privately (Ericka has not). A Web site (The Ingram Organization) is independently maintained; it is devoted to an understanding of the false-memory syndrome and to clearing Paul Ingram's name.

Where Have All the Babies Gone?

Satanic ritual abuse, or SRA, refers to sexual abuse in the context of a satanic ritual. Reports of such bizarre happenings go way back in history, as do many other phenomena dealt with in this book. A witch panic in seventeenth-century Sweden involved the creation of false memories, false allegations of satanic child abuse, and clear psychiatric symptoms.

In recent times, recovered stories of ritualistic abuse of children seemed to surface more frequently in the mid-1980s. I don't recall seeing the term "satanic ritual abuse" prior to that. Indeed, putting "satanic ritual abuse" into a MEDLINE search yields papers only as far back as 1991 (MEDLINE itself goes back over forty years). It was in the 1890s, of course, that Freud made the concept of repressing a memory into an ordinary event. Then there was a time, during the 1980s, when memories uncovered during hypnosis or psychotherapy were believed to always be true. A lot of these memories concerned sexual abuse, even though many studies have shown that at least eighty percent of victims remember the abuse — all too well.

By the mid-1990s, it had become obvious that most of these memories dredged from the subconscious by well-meaning therapists were not so literally true. Maybe they were metaphors for other types of conflicts. Meanwhile, many families were destroyed. In a recent review of a book, *Remembering Trauma* by R. J. McNally (reviewed in the *New England Journal of Medicine* in the November 6, 2003 issue), the points are made that adults nearly always recall documented sexual abuse, and that such recall is never established without independent confirmation.

But for a while, SRA cases became common among psychotherapists, with informal surveys, including one taken by the American Psychological Association, suggesting that ten to fifty percent of therapists were treating at least one SRA patient. I assume this has dwindled lately, and I was unable to find the words "satanic" or "ritual" in the indexes of several recent editions of textbooks of psychiatry, nor any references to SRA in the sections on childhood sexual abuse.

One unifying feature of reported SRA is the inability to come up with any physical evidence in the aftermath of multiple bloody murders, woundings, druggings, bonfires, etc. In a 1991 paper in the journal *Child Abuse and Neglect*, thirty-seven adults who had described such abuse during their childhoods were studied. All or most of the patients reported sexual abuse, witnessing and receiving physical abuse or torture, witnessing animal mutilations or killings, death threats, forced drug usage, witnessing and being forced to participate in human adult and infant sacrifices, forced cannibalism, and marriage to Satan. The authors take a neutral stand on the reality issue.

One of these thirty-seven patients described a ritual where her baby was dismembered and consumed. She then informed the rest of the family that the child had suffered a crib death. In an attempt to verify this, a brother was contacted; he knew of the pregnancy and some sort of "funeral" held at the home, although he never saw the baby. The hospital in which the infant was supposed to have been born had no record of its birth. The state's Bureau of Vital Statistics also had no record of either this birth or death.

As for me, I find it impossible to believe that significant numbers of American babies vanish, unbeknownst to society, leaving behind neither birth certificates, blood, nor bones.

Same Show, Many Viewers

What renders SRA interesting, in a book on unexplained phenomena, is the widespread and sometimes simultaneous nature of the outbreaks, as well as the similarities in the victims' descriptions of the events and circumstances. There is almost a legitimate presumption that all these people read the same book or saw the same movie or TV show (or their therapists did) and, although they've forgotten all about it, this is what informs their SRA accounts now and makes them all similar. Some researchers have found historical SRA panoramas that existed prior to the Inquisition, with similarities to the present time. Professor of pediatrics and psychiatry Frank W. Putnam, at the National Institutes of Mental Health, reviewed, in the same issue of *Child Abuse and Neglect*, the study of the thirty-seven adults reporting SRA. He believes that such historical accounts are not accurate, and cites medieval scholars who find no evidence of satanic cults' existence during those times. Putnam also feels that rumors, urban legends, and folk tales can disseminate rapidly through society.

Walter C. Young, the psychiatrist at the National Center for the Treatment of Dissociative Disorders who was the lead author of the reviewed study, isn't so sure. He is struck by his thirty-seven patients' similar experiences, despite coming from diverse areas and treatment locations, and having minimal contact with each other. Ph.D. psychologist Frank Leavitt at Rush Medical College in Chicago administered word-association tests to SRA and non-SRA patients and concluded that "an experience base is shared by individuals reporting SRA that is not found in individuals who do not report satanic abuse (even if they report sexual abuse)." Leavitt also believes that SRA patients share common knowledge despite their wide geographic separation.

It is this commonality of memory that led Carl Jung to believe in a collective unconscious. Are SRA scenarios somehow embedded into an instinctive human memory base? The "how," not to mention the "why," isn't obvious, but neither is it clear why diverse individuals can report similar bizarre experiences. The absence of any physical traces left behind from the rituals makes it clear that these didn't literally happen; but why would so many people, from different walks of life, share these recollections? And why can't they be convinced that the actual satanic orgies never took place?

Let's look at what kind of person, psychiatrically speaking, reports SRA. Going back to Leavitt's study, which was published in 1998 in the *Journal of Clinical Psychology,* three groups of in-hospital psychiatric patients were compared: those who had reported sexual abuse (non-satanic), those who had reported SRA, and patients from a general psychiatric unit. A word-association test, which uses responses to single words to glimpse conscious and unconscious meanderings of the mind, was administered to all three groups. For example, the word "table" might normally elicit a response of "chair." But if a patient had been sexually abused on a table, even as a child, the response might be "scary" or "violence."

Sexually abused (but non-SRA) patients and general psychiatric patients were similar in their word associations. SRA experiencers were different. They were less likely to come up with normal-type replies and more likely to have satanic-type connections (like responding to the word "circle" with associations like "chanting" or "cult," as opposed to "ball" or "square"). Leavitt and co-author psychologist Susan Labott find that there is a unique pattern of satanic word associations exhibited by SRA patients that is different from the responses of other psychiatric patients, even those who were sexually abused. What's more, they don't feel that these associations were planted by well-meaning therapists, as the patients came from diverse settings and locations; they also believe that some of the associations are subtle and not likely to have occurred from memory "contamination." As for media influences—magazines, movies, and TV—the authors feel that everyone is exposed to these, including the other psychiatric patients who did not answer the test words with satanic references.

In an earlier paper (1994), Leavitt screened SRA and sexually traumatized (without SRA) patients with the dissociative experiences scale mentioned in the NDE chapter. A score of more than thirty is consistent with a dissociative disorder.[8] That chapter's near-death experiencers averaged eleven on this test.

---

8 Dissociative disorders were described in chapter 7, under the subheading "I Am Not Myself," and again in chapter 9, under the subheading "The Non-Association of Mind and Body."

Now Leavitt administered it to his two groups. The abused, non-SRA group averaged thirty-six, indicating some ability to dissociate one's perceived self from reality. But the SRA patients averaged fifty, a high score often seen in multiple personality disorders.

The Three (or More) Faces of Eve

Multiple personality disorder, known as MPD (an astounding number of medical diagnoses can be boiled down to three letters), is a psychiatric condition that some feel is extremely rare and others feel is extremely under-recognized. In epidemiologic studies, between 0.5 percent and 3 percent of patients admitted to psychiatric hospitals meet the diagnostic criteria for this curious affliction, currently classified as dissociative identity disorder (DID) and considered the most serious of the dissociative disorders.

Most MPD patients are women; they tend to be well educated and upper middle class. There is a sense that men with this problem become wards of the criminal justice system rather than of the mental health establishment, and are thus under-reported in clinical series. The young, ghost-possessed London man in a prior chapter comes to mind. Possession states are considered a different variation of dissociative disorder, but I can see how the ghost-directed behavior might qualify as another "personality."

There are some data to suggest that MPD can be hereditary. The condition is often compounded by other symptoms, like moodiness, anxiety, eating disorders, insomnia, and suicide attempts. It is similar to, and can be confused with, borderline personality disorder, which is a different psychiatric classification. A traumatic event, usually in childhood, is believed to precipitate

MPD, which then becomes a defense mechanism to shield the experience by attributing it to another self, not really you. If you hypnotize easily, you may be more susceptible. Some forms of epilepsy, in theory, can cause similar symptoms.

Two or more distinct personalities are required for the diagnosis of MPD; an average patient may have five or ten (think Sally Field in *Sybil*). These must take control of the person's behavior, and there must be no memory within each personality of what happens in the other incarnations. Sometimes there is a "dominant" personality that does retain memory of all the other personae.

I have a patient with MPD. Years ago, she volunteered this information to me, in the context of why I couldn't control her diabetes. Despite my raising her insulin dosage, her blood sugar never went down. Then she let me in on why: She had multiple personalities, many of whom were *not* diabetic (and wouldn't be taking insulin). The medical advice I dispensed in the office would not be relevant at other times, to other selves. Usually we call this noncompliance, but hers was a special case. She also told me, more recently, that each personality has no memory of the others. Her life experiences, therefore, are personality-specific. It's like different users logging on, each with their own password, to the same computer, whose hard drive no one can locate. (Remember, the brain's memories cannot be localized.)

Could the Ingram family be seen as having multiple personalities, one straight and one satanic, each with no connection to or memory of the others? To the extent that the second, satanic-experiencing, personality is "distinct," yes. Certainly the lapses, during questioning, into the hypnotic, trance-like states described in Wright's *New Yorker* articles qualify as some sort of clinical dissociation. Indiana University psychiatrist Philip M. Coons studied twenty-nine patients attending a dissociative disorders clinic who had reported satanic ritual abuse. Twenty-two of them had MPD as well. There is likely much overlap between SRA and MPD. Some observers feel that all patients who report SRA also have MPD. Coons tried to corroborate the abuse stories by interviewing relatives and examining old records; in no case could the reports be verified.

MPD may be falling out of favor as a psychiatric diagnosis. In a 1999 paper in the *American Journal of Psychiatry*, Harrison Pope, one of the authors of the lycanthropy account, assessed attitudes of American psychiatrists towards MPD/DID. Via questionnaires, Pope concluded that there wasn't much consensus about the diagnosis or validity of this syndrome. In a more scathing review in the *Canadian Journal of Psychiatry* in the fall of 2004, the authors feel that these diagnoses are illogical, not clearly diagnosable, not obviously linked to traumas, and to an extent fostered by health care professionals who look for MPD. The title of the two-part dissertation was "The Persistence of Folly."

Regardless of the label's validity, the medical profession is usually the first port of call for individuals and families disrupted and destroyed by intrusions of strange memories and altered personalities and behaviors. Whatever we call our patients, we still have to treat them; in the case of MPD, we haven't been hugely successful.

Again, where do memories come from? From life experience, of course. From a collective unconscious, perhaps. From dreams? "When Dreams Become Reality" was a paper published in the journal *Consciousness and Cognition* in 1996, by psychologists Giuliana A. L. Mazzoni of the University of

Florence, Italy, and Elizabeth F. Loftus of the University of Washington in Seattle. They recruited subjects in their early twenties who could usually remember their dreams. The psychologists created lists of words, some taken from dream content, some not, and subjects were tested as to the source of these words. The people mistook their own dream words with those on the other, non-dream, list "at a very high rate," suggesting that dream elements can easily be remembered as reality. The authors further conclude that "personal dream material seems to have a special quality in terms of its ability to 'become' memory."

Can well-meaning therapists implant memories, just by suggestion to susceptible people that these may be real? Professor of psychology Nicholas P. Spanos published, in 1994, "The Social Construction of Memories," a review of research on odd, evoked memories such as SRA. Spanos believes that a hypnotherapist (many of these memories emerge under hypnosis) can get patients to "recall" things by suggesting to them that certain events may have actually occurred. MPD patients tend to be easily hypnotizable, suggestible folks, and Spanos notes that by the mid-1980s, twenty-five percent of these patients, in therapy, had recovered SRA memories, and that by 1992 this was as high as eighty percent. There is a sense of "seek and ye shall find," and a question as to whether such thoughts were already there, awaiting detection, or were "put in" by the therapist. How easy is it to convince people that they've experienced an inherently bizarre, detailed ritual, anyway? Can some people be *that* suggestible?

Spanos goes on to note that a minority of psychotherapists seems to see the majority of SRA sufferers, and speculates that their therapy may "play an active role in shaping the ritual abuse 'memories' of their patients." Some hypnotists may provide MPD patients with explicit SRA details and ask if any other of their personalities are familiar with them; these may be leading questions. Spanos cites a 1992 paper by psychologist Richard J. Ofshe, "Inadvertent Hypnosis During Interrogation." Ofshe had been called in to evaluate Paul Ingram. This report effectively summarized his conclusions: that the interrogation itself induced hypnosis and the creation of pseudo-memories in a man who was prone to believing whatever he was told.

Just Following Orders

How pliant are people when told to do something by an authority figure? In a famous experiment done in the early 1960s, psychologist Stanley Milgram tested the limits of obedience to authority. At the behest of a stern-looking "authoritative" researcher in a long white coat, test subjects were directed to deliver painful electric shocks to each other, as part of a "learning experiment." Milgram wanted to see just how much pain one person would inflict upon another, simply because they were directed to do so. (These were actually sham shocks, but the person pushing the buttons didn't know that. The experiment would be considered unethical by today's standards.)

It turned out that almost two-thirds of the subjects would administer severely painful electric shocks just because they were told to do so. Some became obviously uncomfortable in their roles as "punishers" but complied nevertheless. The parallel here is that although Paul Ingram was ordered to remember something, rather than to deliver a painful shock, the basic concept of obedience to authority still applies.

If your belief system allows that the devil walks this earth searching for conscripts, you may take SRA literally. If you are a health care professional who believes in MPD/DID as a valid diagnosis based on a child's defense mechanism, then you must consider why many children have survived concentration camps, floods, wars, famines, physical abuse, and other traumas without developing the syndrome. If you don't agree that MPD is a legitimate diagnosis, then what, exactly, *is* wrong with these people? While most of us don't have "photographic" minds, we can still retain a reasonable sense of what has happened in our lives. But why can some people remember, as manifestly real, events that can never be verified? And why can other people have no memory whatsoever of real life (like failing to remember that they have diabetes), because of identity hops, skips, and jumps? We don't really know.

$\mathcal{T}$welve

Dream On: The Meaning of Dreaming

Great mysteries of the brain still exist. One, already mentioned, concerns the storage of long-term memories. Another is why we sleep. Birds do it, perched on a tree branch. Dolphins do it, half a brain at a time, still swimming. All mammals do it, in some form. A third of our lives is spent sleeping; and to this day, we don't know exactly why.

Sleep is obviously a biologic necessity. Get less of it one day, you'll need more the next. Humans (and animals), if totally sleep-deprived, will die. Slumber may be restful, but no amount of rest or immobility will render it unnecessary. We know some restoration of brain chemistry occurs while we sleep, but this doesn't as yet explain why we need our beauty rest to survive.

To Sleep, Perchance to Dream

In 1953, University of Chicago professor of physiology Nathaniel Kleitman and his graduate student, Eugene Aserinsky, performed an elegantly simple experiment. They awakened subjects whose sleeping eyes were noted to be darting around (periods of eye motility), and found that about three-quarters said they were having a dream. When they awakened subjects whose eyes were relatively still, less than 10 percent reported dreaming. Their publication in the journal *Science* was entitled "Regularly Occurring Periods of Eye Motility, and Concomitant Phenomena, During Sleep." Their work was replicated by others, and the current era of dream-study began: You now more or less knew when someone was dreaming, and when they were not, and you could study them accordingly.

There are some who think that one of the main purposes of sleep is to allow dreams, and REM (rapid eye movement) periods, like sleep itself, also appear to be a physiological mandate. Just about all mammals exhibit REM sleep cycles, and humans and animals deprived of REM sleep (by being awakened at the moment the REM begins) will enter this phase sooner the following night. REM and dreaming are considered "concomitant phenomena," and most observers use REM cycles as evidence of dreaming. We spend about 25 percent of our sleep time in REM; newborns spend 50 percent, the elderly about 18 percent. So why do we dream?

The meaning of the dreams themselves has fascinated us since the beginnings of civilization. In ancient Egyptian and Judeo-Christian cultures, dream scenarios were often believed to have resulted from divine intervention. The Bible contains about seventy dream references. Meanwhile, in Asia, dreaming was seen as an opportunity for the soul to leave the body and roam free. This was also believed in primitive tribal societies, with the additional caveat that the floating soul could visit other sleepers as well. The ancient Greeks straddled both theories, accepting at times a wandering, telepathic soul as well as a divinely implanted message.

A new epoch began in 1900, with the publication of Sigmund Freud's *The Interpretation of Dreams*. This now-famous book sold only 351 copies in its first six years (new ideas plod along slowly). And the idea that dream images might have some meaning of their own, open to interpretation, was in contrast to the ancients' philosophies. Now Freud was saying that dreams were windows to an unconscious mind—itself a new concept—mixing snippets of the day ("day residue") with symbols representing a person's inner conflicts created by what he called "primary process." Dreams could now be seen as fulfillment of wishes, conscious or unconscious, and could be used in a psychotherapeutic process.

Freud's revolutionary way of looking at dreams did not entirely exclude telepathy. New York psychiatrist David Shainberg published a paper in the *American Journal of Psychotherapy* in 1976, "Telepathy in Psychoanalysis: An Instance." Before describing his own experience with a patient, Shainberg cites two Freudian references to telepathy in dreams and psychoanalysis. In one, Freud allows for the possibility that some "occult phenomena" may be real; in the other, he wonders if telepathy may have been "the original archaic method by which individuals understood each other."

A Telepathic Dream

Shainberg's case, involving a patient of his referred to as Martin G., in psychoanalysis for the past four years, unfolded as follows: Dr. Shainberg had just received a call that his own father, who lived some distance away, had been taken to the hospital with symptoms of a possible stroke. The next day, Martin G. came in for a session. While his father's illness was on Shainberg's mind, he did not, of course, mention this to his patient. That night the doctor received several more phone calls, regarding the worsening of his father's condition and the necessity for a test known as an angiogram, which requires the injection of a dye into an artery in the neck. This test disclosed an abnormality in Shainberg Senior, necessitating surgery.

When Martin presented for analysis the next day, he volunteered details of a dream he had had the previous night. It involved a man who needed an operation. Shainberg was present in the dream; something had to be injected into the man's head; blood vessels were exposed; afterward, an urgent surgery was needed. There was also, according to Martin, an unusual quality of emotion in this dream.

Shainberg considered Martin G.'s dream to have been telepathic regarding the events developing at the time with his own father. He cited several references in his paper of similar occurrences between patient and doctor during psychoanalysis. He states that "Many investigators have noted that telepathic communication is common when there is sickness or death in the family of the analyst." While the emotion-charge in the doctor might be perceivable, the details causing it would not; so this phenomenon, if it exists, would be unexplained.

The Dream Machine

Also unexplained is why we *need* to dream. We seem designed for it. Sleep allows dream cycles—usually five per night, each lasting roughly twenty minutes (some can span an hour), with the cycles lengthening toward morning. During these cycles of mental activity, the body's muscles are paralyzed by the brain so we don't literally act out our dream scenes. (Nature thinks of everything.) Occasionally this "sleep paralysis" persists into the zone between sleep and wakefulness, giving one a brief, frightening feeling of lying in bed, being unable to move.

REM sleep seems to have some function in consolidation of memories, and in learning and coping, but there are no consistent data on this. What's more, there are patients with brain injuries or on certain medications who no longer have REM sleep, and they seem quite capable of functioning and learning. While dreaming is usually the province of REM sleep, some dreaming occurs in non-REM periods, and not all REM awakenings are associated with dreams.

There are differences in the brain physiology of REM sleep and dreaming. Mark Solms, professor in neuropsychology at the University of Cape Town, wrote a paper, "Dreaming and REM Sleep are Controlled by Different Mechanisms," in which he notes that the parts of the brain responsible for each state are different and able to function independently of each other. Thus, dreaming can occur without REM, and vice versa. Dreaming is subjective, and, as Solms points out, "there is no generally accepted definition of dreaming." I wonder if some dream-inhibiting brain lesions could sever the capacity to ascertain whether one has been dreaming, rather than removing the dreaming itself. Are rapid eye movements associated with a dream akin to watching a movie, so that REM might indicate observation of the dream, rather than the existence of dreaming itself?

Apropos, in a 1962 paper in the *Archives of General Psychiatry,* "Dream Imagery: Relationship to Rapid Eye Movements of

Sleep," patients were awakened immediately by one researcher upon noting any distinct pattern of eye movement. A second researcher, not told of the specific REM pattern, then asked the patient what they were dreaming about. In one example, a dream of climbing stairs and looking at each step corresponded to up-and-down eye movements of the sleeper. The authors, Columbia University psychiatrist Howard Roffwarg and colleagues, summarize by noting that the dreamer "is almost totally immersed in his dreaming consciousness." They find that emotional stress in the dream translates into quickening of pulse and respiration, while the dreamer's eyes flit about following the action. The paper includes a quote from Lewis Carroll: "We often dream without the least suspicion of unreality."

Solms does conclude that "the biological function of dreaming remains unknown." At a 2003 meeting, he responded to a question about whether dreams were meaningless with the answer "probably not." In a recent (2005) review, "Physiology and Psychology of Dreams," University of Michigan psychologist Alan Eiser reviews many of the "impressive advances" we've made in understanding brain function, but points out that "there are widely differing views concerning how dreams should be seen."

Am I Dreaming?

In the last chapter, I quoted a study, "When Dreams Become Reality," where subjects confused words from their reported dreams with non-dream words selected at random. In a further blurring of the distinction between dreaming and real life (as noted by Solms and Eiser), lesions located in certain parts of the brain cause vivid and frequent dreaming as well as a breakdown of the patient's ability to separate the real from the dreamt. While the mental illness schizophrenia cannot be traced to a specific brain lesion, there is a line of research suggesting that dream processes in these patients can "leak through" into waking life. Their hallucinations can thus be seen as "dreaming while awake." Other research has noted that the more severe is the schizophrenia, the less is the time spent in REM sleep, as if the patients' dreamlike, hallucinatory waking hours somehow satisfy their brains' physiologic need for REM periods.

The dreams of schizophrenics are often quite bizarre. There can be dreams of incest. A twenty-six-year-old schizophrenic woman had a dream in which she gave birth to her younger sister. One might wonder whether members of the Ingram family (in the preceding chapter) had dream-versus-reality issues (remember that a lot of schizophrenics, even with treatment, never come to understand that they are hallucinating). Put another way, "when hallucinations become reality" describes the schizophrenic consciousness.

What has been called the "REM intrusion" theory of schizophrenia postulates that dream activity can erupt into real life. Support for this theory came from the finding that a type of electrical activity around the eyes associated with REM sleep could be found in awake, hallucinating schizophrenics. Another avenue of study finds "florid refractory schizophrenias" that are "treatable variants . . . of narcolepsy." Narcolepsy is an uncommon condition where people can sleep. And sleep. And sleep. It is often genetic, and requires high doses of stimulants to prevent inopportune snoozing. In a 1991 paper, psychiatrist Alan Douglass and colleagues describe five schizophrenic patients who also suffered from narcolepsy; their mental illness improved when their narcolepsy was treated with stimulant drugs. Schizophrenia would not itself be helped by these medications, and the premise was that narcoleptic "sleep intrusion" resembled the delusional world of mental illness. Yet this could be successfully treated as a wake/sleep abnormality rather than as a psychosis. While Douglass's patients would only be a small (up to 7 percent) proportion of currently diagnosed schizophrenics, the concept of overlap of narcolepsy, a sleep disorder, and schizophrenia, a thought disorder, is interesting.

Do the arms of Morpheus sometimes reach out and touch us while we're awake? How solid is the wall between dreams and reality? Not everyone, as we've seen, can tell the difference. How could Dr. Shainberg's patient have a dream that reflected reality? And why are we constructed to dream? It can't be just for the purpose of confusing ourselves. . . .

Thirteen

When I Snap My Fingers . . . Hypnosis

On the morning of Friday, February 17, 1978, in the city of Waterloo in Ontario, Canada, a dental surgeon named Victor Rausch had his gallbladder removed. What made this noteworthy was that no anesthesia was used. No drugs, no gas, no acupuncture, no bullet to bite, no whiskey to swig. Dr. Rausch merely hypnotized himself. The operation, known as a cholecystectomy, was at that time done in an "open" fashion, as opposed to the laparascopic slits that current technology offers. This meant making an eight-inch incision through the abdominal wall, entering the abdominal cavity, cutting out the gallbladder, and sewing it all back up.

What turned out to be the most difficult part of the procedure, from Dr. Rausch's point of view, was getting the hospital and the surgical team to let him try this "insane" idea. (That's the word Rausch used when he published his experience two years later in the *American Journal of Clinical Hypnosis*.)

The dental surgeon's experience with hypnosis came from a stint in the army, during which he employed it with patients for painful and traumatic dental procedures. He was impressed that these patients seemed to heal faster, and with less discomfort, than those treated conventionally.

Rausch began his preparation for this mind-over-matter feat the night before, using relaxation and visualization of the operation itself, and focusing on confidence. Wheeled into the O.R. the next morning, the tension of everyone else — none of whom had any experience with hypnosis — was overwhelming. But the patient assured them that all would be well, and separated himself from the situation by concentrating on music playing only in his mind, specifically Chopin's *Nocturne in E-flat*.

Rausch had not known the surgeon, the O.R. personnel, or the stand-by anesthetist beforehand, and met them only briefly prior to his big day. They assured him that the pain would be unbearable and all-consuming, but they could not deter him.

Victor Rausch's blood pressure shot up as the incision was made, while he felt only "an interesting, flowing sensation throughout my entire body." The pressure returned to normal in a few minutes, and the surgery of an hour and fifteen minutes proceeded uneventfully, with the patient conscious, but feeling "as though I were an observer rather than the patient." Eye contact with the nurses seemed to strengthen him. The surgeon even asked him not to try to control his bleeding, for fear that a vessel that might open up later would be missed by the cautery.

Dr. Rausch acknowledges that only a small percentage of the population, at best, could tolerate major abdominal surgery with nothing beyond hypnosis for anesthesia. He assumes his is the first published report, and suggests "that we keep our intuitive channels wide open and learn to expect the unexpected."

Hypnosis Defined

Not everyone can be hypnotized. A Google search on the percentage of the population that is hypnotizable turned up widely different numbers—from 5 percent to 95 percent! Much of this hinged on how hypnosis was defined. What, exactly, is it? Literally, the word means "sleep." But hypnotized subjects are clearly not sleeping in the usual sense. Let's review some definitions:

- In *Trancework: An Introduction to the Practice of Clinical Hypnosis* (2nd ed., 1990), clinical psychologist Michael Yapko begins by reviewing some past definitions. These include:
  - a natural, altered state of consciousness;
  - a relaxed, hyper-suggestible state;
  - guided daydreaming;
  - a twilight state, halfway between sleep and wakefulness.

Yapko also practices therapeutic hypnosis, and he feels that these descriptions only see the process from the subject's point of view. Since Yapko believes hypnosis to be interactive—a series of communications between therapist and patient—he uses the term "influential communication" to define the state.

- *A History of Medical Hypnosis in Psychiatric Clinics of North America* (1994) traces the use of suggestion, sometimes accompanied by ritual or fanfare, as a means of improving health dating back to antiquity, adding: "However these events come to pass, they are mediated through the intimate connection between the sufferer and the healer."

- In *The Practice of Hypnotism* (2nd ed., 2000), hypnotherapist Andre M. Weitzenhoffer introduces hypnosis "as the label for a peculiar state or condition that can presumably be brought about in some human beings." He sees present-day hypnosis as a "suggested effect," and its practice as both a science and an art. In a later chapter, Weitzenhoffer, who had degrees in physics, mathematics, and biology in addition to psychology, views hypnosis "as a state of consciousness characteristically associated with suggestibility."

- A 1999 review of hypnosis in the *British Medical Journal* defines it as "the induction of a deeply relaxed state, with increased suggestibility and suspension of critical faculties."

- A recent edition of a textbook of psychiatry (*Synopsis of Psychiatry,* 9th ed., 2003) presents the definitions according to three prominent practitioners:

  - a state of heightened focal concentration and receptivity;
  - a condition in which a person can respond to appropriate suggestions by experiencing altered perceptions, memory, or mood;
  - a free period in which individuality can flourish.

The last statement is from psychiatrist Milton Erickson, perhaps the best-known and most innovative hypnotherapist of the mid- and latter twentieth century. (Erickson was famous for the creative and outrageous ways in which he could affect patients' behavior. Once, treating a couple whose problem was that they were both bedwetters, he advised them, when bedtime arrived, to get in the bed and urinate into it. Then they were to go to sleep in their sodden bedding. Very quickly, the problem resolved.)

The textbook adds that hypnosis may involve a sense of involuntariness and automatic movements, where suggested perceptions can replace ordinary ones. Elements of trance may include an altered state of consciousness, a dissociative state, or an ability to regress. Alterations in perception, memory, and mood may be evident.

The textbook also defines three levels of a trance state, which a properly hypnotized subject enters. Light trance brings on relaxation of muscles, a weightlessness of the arms, and a gentle, numb feeling. Medium trance involves diminished pain perception and partial or complete amnesia for the events during the session. And heavy trance induces deep anesthesia and hallucinations. Distortions of time, reminiscent of dreaming, occur at all levels, but are greatest in the deepest state.

In Weitzenhoffer's book, the point is made that all hypnosis is essentially trance, but not all trances are hypnotic. The difference is that true hypnosis generally requires two people (hypnotist and subject); they communicate; the hypnotist acquires the power of suggestion. While a phenomenon of self-hypnosis exists, Weitzenhoffer feels that it is vaguely defined, overlaps with positive thinking, or employs a not-physically-present hypnotist via imagination or tape recording.

The gist seems to be that classical hypnosis, like sex, tea, or the tango, can be experienced alone, but is better served by the presence of another person. On the other hand, once taught self-hypnosis by a therapist, patients may continue to treat themselves.

Going Under

Whatever this state is, how easily can you be transported into it? In other words, how hypnotizable are you? Scales to measure hypnotic susceptibility have been in use since the nineteenth century. Many currently exist; and in medicine, when there are many ways of doing something, you can be sure that no single way is clearly superior. One commonly used instrument is the Stanford Scale (there are a number of variations of it), developed in part by Weitzenhoffer. It consists of about a dozen hypnotic parameters, and includes things as simple as whether or not the eyes close spontaneously, or as complex as whether age regression occurs. Another is the eye-roll test, which is a physical measurement. The patient is asked to look up, only with the eyes. Then, eyes upward to the max, he or she is asked to roll the eyelids downward, over the eyes. If properly accomplished, only the whites of the eyes show, ghoulishly. The textbook considers the eye-roll "a presumptive measure of biologic ability to experience dissociation." The implication is that dissociation and hypnosis, particularly in its deeper forms, have a lot in common.

Ironically, Victor Rausch would not have been considered a very good subject by the eye-roll test. In hypnosis, the art and the science, like newlyweds, are presently inseparable.

These scales, and others, can also be used to grade depth of hypnosis. The above-mentioned trance levels are scored, with additional items. One of these is somnambulism—literally, "sleepwalking"—which is considered a facet of heavier hypnotic states. Sleepwalking itself is common, particularly in children, and occurs during non-REM sleep. While psychiatrists don't consider it a form of dissociation, a sleepwalker and a person in a dissociative state have much in common, including an amnesia of the events transpiring, and being observably "not themselves." Weitzenhoffer considers hypnotic somnambulism to be relatively rare and differentiates it from "classical" hypnosis.

Regardless of how hypnosis is defined, or how profound the trance is, there are no objective, physiological measurements that are unique to the state. Brain waves (electroencephalogram, or EEG) are basically the same as when you're awake. Occasionally, subtle EEG changes have been reported, but without consistency or smoking-gun clarity.

Recently, positron emission tomography (PET scans, in the vernacular), which measure regional blood flow and elucidate areas where the brain is active, have shown that the brain seems to perceive what the hypnotist suggests. If the hypnotist suggests that black-and-white pictures are really color pictures, they register in the "color" area of the brain's visual cortex. Hypnotically suggested sounds register as real; imagined sounds do not.

That latter tidbit comes from a 1998 work: "Where the Imaginal Appears Real: A PET Study of Auditory Hallucinations." Volunteers in their early twenties who were easily hypnotizable were divided into two groups. This was not a random separation; one group had the ability to actually hallucinate, if asked to do so, under hypnosis. The authors estimate that only about four percent of highly hypnotizable subjects can do this; these were designated "hallucinators." The other group were "nonhallucinators." The hallucinators' brains had more energetic auditory responses even to normal hearing, suggesting some baseline difference in how their minds processed sounds.

For the experiment, all subjects were hypnotized, and then they listened to a two-and-a-half-minute tape recording of a voice repeating a phrase over and over. "Normal" hearing consisted of just listening to the tape. Imagined hearing consisted of asking the subjects to imagine they were hearing the tape (both groups could do this), without the recorder being turned on again. Hallucinated hearing was obtained by asking the hallucinators to do their thing, and then clicking on the recorder, as if to play the tape, followed by silence. Afterwards, the participants evaluated the sounds they heard, as "external" (hallucinated) or "inside their own heads" (imagined).

Hallucinated sounds produced PET responses similar to those of ordinary hearing; imagined sounds did not. The non-hallucinators' brains did not "hear" mind-produced sounds, as far as the PET scanner was concerned. The implication is that some peoples' brains, at some times, may perceive unreal sounds as real. The authors feel that the auditory hallucinations of schizophrenics share a similar mechanism, and cite studies showing similar brain-site activation during psychotic hallucinations.

(Interestingly, true schizophrenic hallucinations are perceived as external. When a patient describes a voice as originating inside his or her own head, that's technically considered a pseudohallucination. According to the above research, a PET scan could tell the difference.)

It should be added that a flurry of subsequent studies on how schizophrenics' brains perceive auditory hallucinations, using techniques that indicate sites of brain activity (via PET or functional MRI scans), have been a bit contradictory and inconclusive.

While a PET scan may say something about how a hypnotic brain reacts, it does not indicate whether a given person is really hypnotized. There are some, in fact, who question the very existence of a true hypnotic state. In a 1981 paper in *Psychiatry*, "Was I Hypnotized?: A Social Psychological Analysis of Hypnotic Depth Reports," the authors feel that a patient's perception of being hypnotized may reflect the context of the questioning and his or her preconceived ideas about the process, "rather than accurately reflecting a unique state of the person."

Real or not, some strange things happen to the hypnotized. As shown in the example at the beginning of this chapter, enough anesthesia can be produced to perform surgery. People can have no memory of what went on, particularly if the therapist suggests to them that they won't remember. How can you lose your memory of something, simply by being told to forget about it? It happens; I just can't say that I understand how. Other times, hypnosis has been used to enhance memory, although it's not always clear whether these memories are accurate.

Then there's age regression. Certain "highly susceptible" subjects can be taken back to their childhoods, and they will be seen acting and sounding like a child, describing things from a child's point of view. I once attended a hypnotherapist's demonstration at my hospital where a woman, who was a suitable subject and had worked with the therapist before, was quickly regressed before an audience of physicians. To my eye, she could have been acting, but I assumed that she and her hypnotherapist did not come to our hospital to play games.

Early in the twentieth century, questions were raised as to the validity of hypnotic regression. Was it actual, or a re-enactment based on a patient's concept of childhood combined with suggestibility? In the 1930s, two experiments were done. Both employed intelligence tests administered to hypnotized, regressed subjects, who then performed only at grade level for their stage of regression. In the second of these studies, adults were taken back to ages four, six, and ten. Their intelligence and behavior during the tests were appropriate for their "age."

In a 1948 study, regression to infancy produced neurologic reflexes seen only in infants. In 1952, a symposium presented patients whose handwritings and vocabularies regressed in parallel with their ages. There was even knowledge of the correct day of the week for events during the period to which the subject was spirited back in time. The textbook considers these phenomena "controversial," but acknowledges that some of the material may be useful in therapy.

A Little History

However it's defined, hypnosis, or something like it, has been around for ages. It wasn't always called hypnosis. In his 1948 book, *Medical Hypnosis*, assistant professor of psychiatry Lewis Wolberg begins with a historical note, referring to hypnosis as "one of the oldest of the medical arts." In ancient Egypt and Persia, trance states were felt to be of a divine nature. With the establishment of Christianity, however, trances were considered witchcraft, and anything of the sort went underground.

And then along came Austrian physician Anton Mesmer. In 1766, he presented a thesis to the faculty at the University of Vienna claiming that some sort of universal fluid or invisible gas permeated the universe and all things. Man and the planets were thus interconnected, similarly to the way gravity binds the solar system; and what's more, human will could manipulate or redirect this force, as could properly placed magnets. He ultimately named this force "animal magnetism."

Mesmer believed he and others could channel this energy to effect healing. Often the patient was brought into a sort of trance and awoke healthy. Mesmer emphasized the importance of rapport between "magnetizer" and subject, in a way reminiscent of current concepts of hypnosis. Mesmer was also charismatic, flamboyant, mysterious, and theatric, and soon ran afoul of the authorities. He was run out of Vienna to Paris, where in 1784 King Louis XVI appointed a commission, headed by Benjamin Franklin, to evaluate his methods and claims.

The Franklin commission concluded that animal magnetism did not exist, and that any improvements in illness could be accounted for by imagination, imitation, and touch. A 2002 paper in the *International Journal of Clinical Hypnosis* remarked that imagination is part of the hypnotic process, regardless of magnetism's existence. Mesmer was discredited and his popularity waned, but words like "mesmerized" in our lexicon attest to his mark on history.

One of Mesmer's disciples, the Marquis de Puysegur, observed and described three cardinal features of what is now known as hypnosis: The "magnetized" subject was only attentive to the "magnetizer" (and to nothing else); the subject was extremely suggestible; the subject had no memory of events during the trance. Puysegur was a nobleman, and he entranced a young servant on his estate who then fell into a strange type of sleep, during which he was ambulatory and hyperalert. He spoke freely and confided family problems that had hitherto been unspoken. Awakened, he had no recollection of what had happened. Puysegur labeled this "artificial somnambulism."

Puysegur believed, as did Mesmer, that the operator's faith in an ability to cure was essential to the process. Positive thinking by practitioner and patient has always been an element of medical care, and that's no less true today. That's why the placebo effect—the improvement reported after mock therapy—tends to be 40 percent, whether you're treating angina, eczyma, or the common cold.

In the early 1800s, there emerged a sense that mesmerism was actually a neurophysiological variant of sleep. That's when it became "hypnosis." A proponent of this theory, James Braid, believed that an intelligent secondary consciousness must exist, which could be unmasked by the hypnotic process.

As the nineteenth century proceeded, many reports came in—particularly from Britain and India—of surgical procedures, some major, performed with only hypnosis for anesthesia. According to Wolberg's book, in 1891 the British Medical Association issued an opinion that "as a therapeutic agent, hypnotism is frequently effective in relieving pain, procuring sleep and alleviating many functional ailments."

In the 1880s, Josef Breuer, a colleague of Sigmund Freud, was treating a young woman known as Anna O. for a multitude of physical and mental problems. He diagnosed her as a hysteric. One symptom she developed was an inability to swallow water. On hot days, she had to quench her thirst with melons and fruit. Under hypnosis, she angrily recounted an incident where she had watched a dog drink water out of a glass, which struck her as disgusting. After venting, she asked for a glass of water, awakened while drinking it, and never had the problem again. This was considered the first case of psychoanalysis—where an unconscious memory causing a symptom was brought to the surface, resulting in the symptom's disappearance. Freud, just beginning his career, found this case fascinating; the rest is history.

In *A History of Medical Hypnosis* (mentioned earlier), authors Joy Dana Riskin and Fred Frankel, of the Harvard Medical School Department of Psychiatry, feel that the domain of modern hypnosis contains elements of suggestion, which they see as Mesmer's legacy, as well as aspects of dissociation, which they attribute to the work of Puyseger and Pierre Janet. The Frenchman Janet was a physician, psychiatrist, and philosopher, and believed that hypnosis and hysteria were mentally similar.

The "History" also remarks that a given individual's hypnotizablity is consistent over time, and that it correlates with certain types of problems. Patients with phobias, eating disorders, post-traumatic stress disorder, and multiple personality disorder tend to be good hypnotic subjects. MPD is also associated with dissociative tendencies, suggesting that hypnosis may be relevant in understanding and treating multiple personalities.

Hypnosis in Medicine

Irritable bowel syndrome afflicts about 15 percent of the American population. Somewhere between 30 and 70 percent of visits to gastroenterologists in the United States are for IBS, depending on whose figures you use. IBS tends to be recurrent, annoying, and painful, and there is no consistently helpful treatment. Pills are dispensed. Diets are suggested. Tests are negative and are only useful to rule out other things.

A unifying feature of the disease is a sensitivity of the colon, or large intestine, to pressure. In a classic experiment, published in the *Lancet* in 1980, a balloon inflated in varying parts of the colon at measurable, equivalent pressures caused more pain over a wider area in IBS patients than in nonafflicted controls. It was as if the patients' colons were overwired with nerve connections, and were thus extra-sensitive.

In 1984, the *Lancet* published a "Controlled Trial of Hypnotherapy in the Treatment of Severe Refractory Irritable-Bowel Syndrome." Thirty IBS patients were randomly assigned to psychotherapy or hypnotherapy. Psychotherapy had some success, with a small improvement in some symptoms. But hypnotherapy patients "showed a dramatic improvement in all features," and were notably better served than the other group.

Three months later, none of the hypnotherapy-treated patients had relapsed. Gastroenterologist Peter Whorwell, lead author of the study, which was done in South Manchester in Britain, later published an eighteen-month follow-up of the patients. All remained in remission. Two had had exacerbations, which were effectively treated with a single additional hypnotherapy session. Reporting on an additional thirty-five IBS patients, Dr. Whorwell remarked that patients with typical IBS who were under age fifty had 100 percent response rates. In a 2003 study at the same institution, the majority of 204 patients treated with hypnotherapy for IBS were better five years later, and needed fewer consultations and medications. Treatment consisted of twelve sessions, over three months, of "gut-directed" therapy, aimed at having patients "visualize" their intestines to gain some measure of control.

On this side of the pond, IBS hypnotherapy was investigated at the University of North Carolina in 2002. Patients felt better and had less discomfort, although physiological parameters measured, such as rectal pain thresholds for balloon inflation, did not change. Nevertheless, the authors were sufficiently impressed with the results that they are trying, via a Web site, to make hypnotherapy for IBS more widely available.

Hypnosis has many other medical uses, and these were reviewed by physician James H. Stewart in the April 2005 issue of the *Mayo Clinic Proceedings*. Stewart's definition of hypnosis reflects those I mentioned earlier, and while Stewart makes no attempt to explain how suggested niceties translate into bodily health, he is willing to say that "If positive suggestions for change are accepted by the mind, any physiological changes that follow defy explanation by contemporary medicine. . . ."

Stewart goes over the published clinical trials of hypnosis. The list is extensive, so we'll just hit the highlights:

- **Allergy.** Hypnotizable patients could be "taught" to react on one arm but not the other when scratched with something to which they were allergic.

- **Pain relief.** Hypnosis has a history of use for pain; of interest is that it appears different from acupuncture. You don't need to be hypnotizable to respond to acupuncture. Also, the use of a drug that blocks the brain's endorphins (a sort of natural morphine) impedes the pain-relieving effects of acupuncture, but not of hypnosis.

- **Anesthesia.** Hypnosis was used as a sole anesthetic agent back in the pre-chloroform era; nowadays it has been used as an adjunct to conscious sedation (where drugs render the patient conscious but dreamy) for procedures that might ordinarily require general anesthesia (like removal of the thyroid, or tubal ligation).

- **Warts.** These fickle creatures are caused by a live virus and have minds of their own. Spontaneous clearing is not infrequent, so an experiment was designed thusly: Fourteen patients with bilateral warts were given suggestions to clear one side only. Ten of the patients could be brought into moderate-depth hypnosis. Of these ten, nine cleared the warts only on the suggested side!

- **Headache.** Administered hypnosis, as well as teaching patients to do self-hypnosis, has had some success.

- **Stopping smoking or overeating.** Some successes, less than dramatic. Nothing deals all that well, particularly over the long term, with these entities.

- **Asthma.** Some success, particularly in younger and more hypnotizable people.

- **Cancer.** Hypnosis and the teaching of self-hypnosis have been helpful in lessening the nausea and vomiting caused by chemotherapy in children.

- **Erectile dysfunction.** One experienced practitioner reported an 88 percent success rate with almost three thousand patients.

- **Urinary incontinence.** One trial cured the majority of women in one month.

All of these treatments require a skilled practitioner and a hypnotizable patient. This is a drawback that limits the usefulness of hypnosis in the all-too-real world.

Hypnosis and ESP

Lastly, hypnosis has been used to enhance ESP. Psychologist Thelma Moss, who co-authored the "Study of a Psychic" discussed in chapter 3, wrote an earlier paper (1970), "Hypnosis and ESP: A Controlled Experiment." Using pairs of volunteers, a "transmitter" was shown emotionally charged material with positive or negative content, while a "receiver," at a distance, had to sense which type it was. Hypnosis of one pair member, usually the receiver, was associated with more correct answers. While the statistical results would not be likely to convert a skeptic, they were also not likely to have occurred by chance. Moss cites other work on ESP facilitation by hypnosis.

Modern practitioners claim that you've experienced a form of hypnosis if you've driven your car along monotonously and don't remember passing a few exits. Can that really be the same phenomenon that cures warts, allows you to undergo major surgery without anesthesia, or takes you back to your childhood? "Hypnosis" obviously means different things to different observers; while it defies precise, objective definition, it has endured in various forms for ages, and is not likely to go away soon.

Fourteen

Xenoglossy: Speaking in Tongues, Coherently

In Mt. Orab, Ohio, on May 10, 1970, the Reverend Carroll Jay, an ordained minister of the United Methodist Church, hypnotized his forty-seven-year-old wife, Dolores. The reverend was a serious amateur hypnotist, so there was nothing unusual about this situation. Dolores had a backache. The hypnosis, it was hoped, could afford her some relief from pain. During this session, when her husband asked her if she still had pain, Dolores replied "nein"—the German word for "no."

The problem was that neither of them spoke German. Intrigued, Reverend Jay re-hypnotized his wife three days later and tried to expand upon what had happened. Encouraged to speak German, in trance, she did. The minister asked the questions in English; Dolores replied largely in German, and in the voice of a young child. Since he could not understand her, Carroll found some friends who could speak

German and had them listen to the sessions, which he had taped.

Gretchen

Dolores spoke German, under hypnosis, responsively, meaning she answered in German whether the query was posed in English or in German (some sessions were attended by German-speakers). Only she wasn't Dolores; she was Gretchen. And the time in which she lived, placed by events of which she spoke, would have been the late nineteenth century.

The phenomenon of age regression under hypnosis was discussed in the previous chapter. Apparently, some subjects can be regressed further — beyond their own lifetimes, into what seems to be a previous life. This is a not-uncommon happenstance with hypnosis, and some clinical hypnosis books even mention it. For example, in *Hypnosis: Questions and Answers* (1986), a chapter is devoted to past-life regression. The author does not object to anyone believing in reincarnation (implied by remembrance of a prior life), but does remark that science has yet to validate such a claim.

"Past lives" evoked under hypnosis have often attracted much public attention and have been the subject of best-sellers. They are less useful for scientific study, as it is known that hypnotized individuals are highly suggestible and try to please their inquisitor, and because details of the times and places of ordinary folk living hundreds of years ago are sparse and not useful for "confirmation." That is why "past lives" emerging during hypnotic states will not be dealt with in this book. And this chapter only examines the speaking of a seemingly never-learned but real language, which cannot be concocted on the spot. While this might imply reincarnation, and has been investigated as such, the linguistic phenomena are more amenable to study.

Suffice it to say that Gretchen's accounts were more or less consistent, including her last name (Gottlieb), the town in which she lived (Eberswalde), and her death—a murder—at about the age of sixteen. Not to mention the fact that she could speak German, and even used some archaic and obscure words.

The Investigation

Ian Stevenson, M.D., now well into his eighties, is a professor of psychiatry at the University of Virginia in Charlottesville. He holds an endowed chair and has served as chairman of the Department of Psychiatry at the University's medical school. He has an interest in studying accounts suggestive of reincarnation. After a letter from Reverend Jay, about his wife, appeared in a psychic magazine, Stevenson contacted the Jays. His report of "The Case of Gretchen" was published in *The Journal of the American Society for Psychical Research* in 1976. While the *Journal* is not indexed in MEDLINE, Stevenson's credentials and the meticulousness of his work merit its review.

Stevenson referred to the phenomenon of someone speaking a language they presumably never learned as "xenoglossy." (Some use the term "glossolalia" for this, although glossolalia is used more often for "speaking in tongues"—technically, a babble that sounds like language but isn't.) In the case of D. J., as she is referred to in the paper, her answers in German constituted "responsive xenoglossy."

Stevenson speaks German, and first ascertained that D. J. was, in fact, responding in coherent German in her "Gretchen" mode. He then obtained assurances from the couple that neither had ever had any prior knowledge of the language; they even signed affidavits to this effect. Mrs. Jay would eventually take a lie-detector test in New York City, which showed that she believed she was telling the truth about never having learned German.

The focus of the paper is an investigation into whether Dolores Jay could have learned to speak German at some juncture in her past, and perhaps had forgotten about it. She was born in Clarksburg, West Virginia, and at the age of two moved to a neighboring town. Her only German ancestry consisted of two great-great-grandparents on her mother's side, who had died many years before her birth. Stevenson interviewed D. J.'s mother, who told him that she had never heard any family member speak German.

Carroll Jay (C. J.) was from the same area of West Virginia. He and Dolores were high-school sweethearts and married soon after graduation. Stevenson went back to the Clarksburg area where both Jays had grown up and interviewed nineteen relatives and neighbors of Dolores Jay, including her parents and a younger sister. All denied having any family or acquaintances who spoke German. No German books had ever been in the house. Young Dolores could not have toddled off and learned a foreign language unbeknownst to her parents, who kept a close eye on her (the parents also signed affidavits as to the truth of their reports).

Stevenson even found statistics as to the number of German-speaking persons in Harrison County, West Virginia, where the Jays' hometowns were located, but could find no one conversant in this language anywhere near the wandering range of a young, supervised child. Even the schools of Harrison County did not teach German at the time the Jays were enrolled there.

So what are we left with? Stevenson is certain that this Gretchen character can speak German. He does not believe the Jays are trying to commit some type of elaborate fraud, and he visited the area where Dolores grew up, satisfying himself that there was no way she could have picked up German. In conclusion, he sees "no reason to be rushed toward final judgments in this matter," but believes "that responsive xenoglossy derives from *some* paranormal process."

As for the reverend, although he had dabbled in hypnotic regression previously, he had made no attempt to accomplish this with his wife. In fact, C. J. found the idea of reincarnation somewhat incompatible with the teachings of Christianity, nor did he care for the concept of possession, which bespeaks of the devil. The couple also had no involvement with parapsychology or cults. But despite their own bewilderment, the Jays felt that something had transpired that was worthy of scientific study. Their case attracted some notoriety, and an article about it appeared in the *Washington Post* in 1975.

Sharada

Stevenson has reported other cases. In 1979 in the *American Journal of Psychiatry* (which is MEDLINE-indexed), he published "A Case of Secondary Personality with Xenoglossy." This time, hypnosis was not involved. The case was that of a thirty-two-year-old single woman, living in the state of Maharashtra in India, who would periodically undergo some sort of change in her personality.

Ms. A., as she was called, spoke Marathi, her native language . . . until her personality changed. This came on gradually, over several hours. Then she became "Sharada" and spoke fluent

Bengali. Dr. Stevenson and research associate Satwant Pas-
richa, Ph.D., studied Ms. A. and interviewed her during her
normal states. She taught at a university, and at times helped her
mother with housework. She and her family denied any knowledge of the Bengali language, had always lived in Maharashtra,
and had never visited the Bengali region of India.

Like patients with multiple personality disorder, Ms. A. and
Sharada seemed to have no knowledge of the other's personality or its pertinent events. A few Bengali speakers were
enlisted by the family to translate during the Sharada
episodes, which could last anywhere from one day to seven
weeks. Sharada described places and events consistent with
early-nineteenth-century Bengal. Her Bengali was appropriate to that era, and not to the modern language. As
Sharada, she dressed and acted like a married Bengali woman,
was familiar with Bengali foods and cooking, had some familiarity with the area's geography, and related that she had died
from a snake bite.

From his meetings with Mrs. A. and her family, Stevenson is
convinced that "she had no normal knowledge of spoken
Bengali." While one could postulate that Ms. A., as a child,
could have seen a book about Bengali history and culture and
didn't remember it, fluency in a language, Stevenson is quick to
point out, is a skill. One doesn't acquire such a skill in a forgotten afternoon; the professor believes Ms. A.'s Bengali to
have been paranormally acquired.

Stevenson had published an earlier report (1974) in *The
Journal of the American Society for Psychical Research* regarding an
American woman who could speak an unlearned language—
Swedish. Similarly to the Jays, this occurred under hypnosis
performed by the husband. Unlike the Jays, who went public

out of a belief that their experiences might have some scientific value, this couple wished to avoid any limelight, and the report identifies them only by their initials.

Jensen Jacoby

T. E. was a thirty-seven-year-old Jewish housewife in Philadelphia in 1955. Her husband, K. E., was a physician in general practice who occasionally employed medical hypnosis with his patients. During an attempt at age regression, T. E. visualized a scene where old people were being forced into a body of water, ostensibly to drown them. In trance, she felt her head being pushed into the water, and suddenly let out a scream and clutched her head, as if she had been clobbered. She awoke with a headache that persisted for two days, and a sense of a lump on her head.

A week later, K. E. hypnotized and regressed his wife again, with the same result. A similar session a week after that also culminated in the same headache. A month later, a different hypnotist was brought in who regressed the wife to the brink of the "incident" and then suggested to her that she go back in time to ten years before the incident. Then the fun began.

Speaking in a deep, masculine voice, the hypnotized T. E. announced: "I am a man." "His" name was Jensen Jacoby, and he was a Swedish peasant farmer. Jensen spoke in broken English and used some foreign-language phrases that sounded Scandinavian. At subsequent sessions, with K. E. back as hypnotist, the same type of linguistics ensued; but following these sessions, some speakers of Swedish and other Scandinavian languages were present. Then, Jensen spoke almost exclusively in Swedish, although he could reply in a halting English if a question were posed in English. The Swedish speakers thought his

Swedish accent was "excellent" and commented on several specific Swedish words that non-native speakers generally mispronounce but which Jensen handled fluently.

Jensen Jacoby described the life of a peasant farmer, raising livestock, before the industrial revolution. He had no familiarity with modern tools but was acquainted with crops, foods, and types of ships that would have been known in seventeenth-century Sweden. His dialect was also consistent with that era.

Jensen was apparently Christian, but the surname Jacoby was frequent among Jews living in Sweden. Sporadic Jewish immigration to Sweden began during the seventeenth century, but conversion to Lutheranism was a requisite. Jensen was vague about his father's origins; he said his mother came from Norway, and he identified his own wife as "Latvia," which was not a Swedish name.

In one of the sessions, T. E. was regressed once more to the headache that started it all. Jensen was sixty-two now, and was engaged in some sort of battle with enemies who pushed him into water while delivering a severely painful blow to the head, which seems to have killed him.

Stevenson spent about fifty hours with K. E. and T. E., investigating this case. As with the Jays, he focused his attention on any possibility that T. E. could have learned Swedish "normally." He interviewed the housewife's eldest daughter and three members of her childhood family (her mother and two older siblings). T. E.'s parents were immigrants from Odessa, Russia, and had never been to Scandinavia, nor did they know anyone who spoke Swedish. English was the language of the Philadelphia neighborhood in which they settled; the parents occasionally spoke Yiddish, Polish, or Russian in the house, but never any Scandinavian language. At the high school she attended, French, Spanish, and Latin were the foreign languages offered (T. E. took some French).

The Swedish speakers who conversed with "Jensen" confirmed that the language was Swedish, with a fluency beyond mimicry or a few phrases. His vocabulary was well over a hundred words, some of which he introduced before hearing them from the interpreters. His accent was authentic; he did not speak Swedish as an American would.

Stevenson administered language aptitude and psychological tests. T. E. did not show much facility for learning a language; she tested psychologically normal. What's more, if she was hypnotized but not regressed, she demonstrated no knowledge of the Swedish language.

Stevenson could find nothing to suggest that fraud could have been involved. Aside from signed affidavits from T. E. and her mother as to the truthfulness of their statements, and a polygraph test which T. E. passed, there seemed to be no motive, psychological or otherwise, for such an elaborate scheme to be perpetrated. The interviews with the family ruled out what Stevenson calls cryptamnesia—forgetting that one has learned something. Again, conversing in a language is a skill; it takes practice.

This Isn't Normal

So that brings us to non-normal explanations, needed for all three cases. Telepathy? Stevenson considers the possibility that a language could have been learned telepathically, from someone else who spoke it. But he comments in his 1984 book *Unlearned Language*, which discusses the Gretchen and Sharada cases in detail (and makes comparisons to Jensen), that "To speak a language intelligibly, it is not enough just to have a limited vocabulary of words in it; one must be able to understand what someone else says in the language and be able to deploy an appropriate reply in the same language." All three could do this, so telepathy, assuming it even exists, wouldn't account for responsive xenoglossy.

Possession? In an earlier chapter, I described the report of a young Londoner who could see the "ghost" of an old woman coming and then uncontrollably possessing his body. Gretchen and Jensen had to be invoked by hypnotic trance. Sharada was simply a benign personality, not a Mr. Hyde to Ms. A.'s Dr. Jekyll. Gretchen slipped in and out of each personality without remembrance of the other, and without any sense of being "controlled."

Stevenson even considers the possibility of "genetic memory." In animals, this would be called "instinct." A bird "knows" how to build a nest without having to be taught. Do we "know" things like foreign languages via our genes? Not if our current understanding of genetics is correct: What our ancestors learned in life isn't supposed to be encoded into our DNA and passed on.

Comparing the three cases, two were evinced under hypnosis, one was spontaneous. Jensen differed in gender; the other two did not. Sharada was quite fluent in Bengali, while Gretchen and Jensen spoke in a more fragmentary fashion. All three alter personalities died unnaturally: Gretchen and Jensen by murder, Sharada by snakebite.

The uniqueness of Stevenson's work is its thoroughness. He used native speakers to verify that the subjects could converse in a foreign tongue, and published transcriptions of the recorded conversations. He thoroughly picked apart every aspect of their pasts, going back to childhood and schooling, and speaking to friends, family, and neighbors. He has done his best to rule out fraud and forgetfulness, and fully believes in the integrity of the subjects.

Stevenson was unable to historically confirm the places and events in the lives of Gretchen and Jensen. However, in Sharada's case, a family was identified, with the same surname Sharada claimed to have had, that lived in Bengal at about the time of the Indian woman's apparent tenure there. As Sharada, Ms. A. had a detailed knowledge of life in nineteenth-century Bengal, including customs, geography, and foodstuffs, and Stevenson finds it implausible that these facts could all have been gleaned from books.

There have been many other reports of spoutings of "unlearned" languages. Stevenson reviews these in his 1974 introduction to the Sharada case. Some were examples of phrases heard in childhood and long forgotten; these people could not carry on conversations in the language. Of those who could, some cases dated back to the mid-nineteenth century, but Stevenson does not consider these accounts to be sufficiently researched and detailed. In fact, after his first publication on this topic in 1974, he received many letters regarding similar happenings, but the lack of documentation and/or tape recordings of sessions render these only "a catalogue of missed opportunities."

Ian Stevenson believes that these cases provide evidence for some sort of survival of personality after death. I can't claim to understand these phenomena myself, but I am convinced that Stevenson's reportage is accurate, that fraud was not involved, and that there is currently no good explanation of why these events occurred. But we should eventually understand them.

$\mathcal{F}$ifteen

Déjà Vu All Over Again: Children Who Remember Past Lives

In researching the paranormal in medicine, perhaps the strangest and most troubling things one finds are the accounts of young children who remember, with confirmable accuracy, someone else's previous life. The collection of these cases has been largely the life work of psychiatrist Dr. Ian Stevenson (who studied xenoglossy, described in the previous chapter), although other researchers are involved. While some of Stevenson's work has reached MEDLINE publications, much of it has appeared in the non-indexed *Proceedings of the American Society for Psychical Research* and the *Journal of Scientific Exploration,* and details of the cases, along with commentary, can be found in Stevenson's books, the most recent of which is a revised edition (2001) of *Children Who Remember Previous Lives.*

Such a Child

All the stories have basic similarities. Here's an example.[9] In India, in 1950, a ten-year-old boy named Nirmal died at home of smallpox in the town of Kosi Kalan (I'll abbreviate it henceforth as K.K.). Sixteen months later, a male infant named Prakash was born six miles away in the village of Chhatta. When Prakash was about four, he began awakening during the night and running outside, claiming that his name was Nirmal and he wanted to go home. "Home" was K.K. He persisted in asking his family to take him to K.K., until finally, when he was five, they decided to humor him. His uncle first took him on a bus that was actually going away from K.K., but the boy seemed to know the misdirection and insisted that they travel the other way, which they then did. At the child's behest, they went to the shop owned by the Jain family (Nirmal's parents). But the shop was closed, and they gave up and returned to Chhatta. Eventually, the Jain family got wind of this visit.

Prakash often insisted on being called Nirmal, and told his mother that she was not his mother. The family was not amused by their son's behavior, and began punishing him for it, sometimes corporally. Yet he continued to profess vivid memories of Nirmal and his relatives and friends. A few more years passed, and Prakash spoke less of this other life, and began to forget it.

When Prakash was ten, Nirmal's older brother, J. Jain, moved back to K.K. (he had been living some distance away) and heard tell of the boy in Chhatta who claimed to be Nirmal and who had identified J. Jain's father, by name, as his own. A few months later, the father, B. Jain, happened to be in

---

9 In: *Twenty Cases Suggestive of Reincarnation* 2nd ed. 1974. Charlottesville: University Press of Virginia.

Chhatta on business. Curious, he looked up Prakash, who immediately recognized him as "his father." A few days later, some other members of the Jain family came by, including Nirmal's mother and older sister. At the sight of the sister, whom he named correctly, Prakash wept with joy.

The Jains persuaded Prakash's parents to let the boy come visit again. On arrival in K.K., Prakash seemed to know the way to the house, and, entering it, he correctly recognized several relatives and friends of the Jains, as well as parts of the house where Nirmal had lived.

The Jain family accepted and embraced the idea that Prakash was Nirmal reborn. Prakash's folks were less enthused and did their best to discourage their child from visiting K.K. (including, once again, corporal punishment).

Dr. Stevenson began investigating the case in 1961, shortly after the boy's second visit to K.K. Prakash's family was somewhat paranoid, fearing that the Jains wished to adopt their son. However, at subsequent interviews a few years later, this concern had abated, and Dr. Stevenson was able to speak extensively with both families.

As with the studies of xenoglossy, the investigation focused on whether the information acquired by the four-year-old could have come from friends or family, or from a willful attempt at fraud. Stevenson met with both sets of parents and siblings, as well as some friends and neighbors and Prakash himself. Prakash's memories of being Nirmal Jain had faded considerably, but they returned when he was questioned about it or when he visited the town of K.K.

Members of both families denied ever meeting or having knowledge of the other. Being of different sub-castes, it was unlikely that they shared friends. The animosity of Prakash's parents, and the joy Stevenson witnessed on the boy's face when he was in the presence of the Jains, made an elaborate hoax unlikely.

Stevenson tabulated Prakash's remembrances, identifying the family member who provided the information, as well as the one who confirmed it, and added comments. There were thirty-four items in all. Prakash knew the names of neighbors, including one who was alive when Nirmal lived but had since died. He knew that the family owned four shops, and that the shops sold shirts. He picked out Nirmal's older brother in a crowd of people in the Jain house. He identified the room where Nirmal slept and the one in which he died. He recognized the tax collector and the Jains' family physician. Stevenson does not believe all this knowledge was obtained "normally."

Roberta Has Two Mommies

Here's another example.[10] Roberta Morgan was born in Minnesota in 1961. At the age of two and a half, she began to speak of a previous life, and of her "other mommy and daddy." Roberta did not supply another name for herself, but she seemed to have clear images of these other parents, and she often compared Mrs. Morgan to the other woman—and not always favorably.

Roberta's "previous family" lived on a farm not far away, and had horses and dogs. Once when the girl was four, she visited a horse farm and was unusually comfortable around the animals, walking up to the horses and petting them, adding that

10 *Children Who Remember Previous Lives*, rev. ed. Jefferson, North Carolina: Mc Farland & Co. 2001. (Stevenson has slightly altered the names used in this book).

she had "been on horses lots of times." She requested toys like the ones she used to have. Sometimes she joined parental conversations, seeming versed in subjects that she shouldn't have known anything about.

One time, when the family was out driving, they passed a dirt road and Roberta asked them to turn, saying the farm was down that road. They ignored her. Her parents were Christian, and reincarnation was not part of their belief system. Soon, the girl's carryings-on got on Mrs. Morgan's nerves, and recollections of life on the farm brought spankings; the spontaneity ceased.

In 1971, Mrs. Morgan heard about the work of Ian Stevenson, and telephoned him. He met with her and interviewed her extensively. She supplied the above information (her daughter had by now completely forgotten it). After much consideration, Mrs. Morgan had had a change of heart, and now regretted having stifled her daughter's memories. For reasons Stevenson never fully understood, Mrs. Morgan never did look for that dirt road again.

Susan and Her Sister

Another American case was that of a child in Idaho named Susan Eastland.[11] The Eastlands, also Christian, did not subscribe to reincarnation. At about two years of age, Susan appeared to make references to her older sister, Winnie, who had been hit by a car and killed three years before Susan's birth. Susan repeatedly claimed that she was six years old (Winnie's age at death). Spotting a photograph of the sister,

11 ibid.

Susan announced that this was a picture of her. She knew certain aspects of the sister's routine, and some specific scenarios involving Winnie and who she was with at the time. She remembered (as Winnie) being kissed by a little boy in a bowling alley (the incident had annoyed the Eastlands). At two, according to Stevenson, Susan "could barely scrawl," but she wrote "winni" on the kitchen door with a crayon.

Charlotte Eastland, her mother, learned about Dr. Stevenson's line of research in a magazine and wrote him. After an exchange of letters, he visited her in Idaho in 1969, when Susan was five. Until then, she hadn't told her children (Susan and two older siblings) that she thought Susan might be Winnie reborn; but following the visit, she told the inquisitive children the reason for it. Charlotte continued to attend her church, but, in order to remain a congregant in good standing, kept her family's experiences concealed.

A Catalogue of Cases

Archived at the University of Virginia at Charlottesville are the details of over 2,500 cases like the ones above. About 1,400 were examined personally by Dr. Stevenson; the others by his colleagues. They were collected from around the globe, and they have certain similarities. Some of these are noted in a 1983 paper by Dr. Stevenson in *The Journal of Nervous and Mental Disease:* "American Children Who Claim to Remember Past Lives."

In this work, generalizations that can be made include the mean age at which a child begins making statements (thirty-seven months of age) and ceases to make them (six or seven years old). The children often manifest oddball personality traits that correspond to those of the deceased. There may be relevant phobias, such as a fear of the water in a person whose "previous personality" (Stevenson's term) had drowned. Or cross-dressing may be noted if the prior personality was of the other sex. The recalled lives tended to be those of ordinary, everyday people.

The main thrust of the paper was to compare American children's past-life remembrances with those of similar children in India. These are different cultures, with different beliefs. Gallup polls have the percentage of Americans believing in reincarnation at about 25 percent, while Hindus, particularly in northern India, largely accept person-to-person reincarnation. It is possible that a family's belief system could affect a child's enthusiasm for "coming forward."

When a child's pronouncements can be corroborated by finding records or family members of the person whom the child "remembers," the case is deemed "solved." When no such individual can be located, it is deemed "unsolved." One difference between the children from America and those from India is the percentage of solved cases. Among 266 cases from India, 77 percent were considered solved, whereas in the U.S. this figure was only 20 percent for the seventy-nine cases studied. In the examples above, that of Prakash/Nirmal and Susan/Winnie would be recorded as solved, while that of Roberta would go down as unsolved.

Other differences: Of the solved cases in the U.S., the child's persona usually corresponded to that of a deceased family member. In India, this was true only 16 percent of the time; most Indian cases involved an unrelated person living anywhere from six to seventy miles away. Only about a third of the American kids knew the name of the person they claimed to be, whereas three-quarters of the Indian children named their alter-ego selves.

One troubling thing that both groups shared: The majority of the deaths that preceded the "reborn" child were violent. Indian children tended to identify how the demise occurred, while Americans did not (for cases within a family, these details would of course be available, as in the case of Susan Eastland). Phobias in the child, as I mentioned, seemed to correspond to the method of death.

In the paper, Stevenson discusses the possibilities of childhood fantasies or imaginary friends accounting for some of the data. Fantasy could be involved in some cases, but he notes that parents often do not warmly receive their children's previous life musings, so such a fantasy creates conflict rather than comfort. And imaginary playmates are living, not previously deceased.

Stevenson addresses the issue of another person's life details trickling into a family where they might have been subconsciously available to the child. He cites several cases from India where there was considerable mileage between the two involved families, and where a written record—later verifiable—was made of the child's comments before the two families had ever met. (In India, where reincarnation has acceptability, it is not uncommon for the two families related in this most unusual way to get together.)

Lastly, Stevenson wishes to alert psychiatrists and primary care physicians to the possibility that such a case could come to their attention. Neither the child nor the family need be considered psychotic; reporting of cases for further study may be warranted. Stevenson assumes that many cases go unreported or unrecognized.

Who Are These Children, Anyway?

Dr. Erlandur Haraldsson, now a professor emeritus in the faculty of social science at the University of Iceland, published a paper in 1995, "Personality and Abilities of Children Claiming Previous-Life Memories," in *The Journal of Nervous and Mental Disease.* He investigated, in detail, twenty-three new cases in Sri Lanka. The circumstances of these cases were quite similar to the ones Stevenson had evaluated.

Data collection may be different in Sri Lanka than it might be at, say, Harvard Medical School. Haraldsson, an interpreter, a Sri Lankan psychologist, and their rental-van driver paid unannounced calls to each subject at home or at school. (Most of the families had already been interviewed by a team member.) To compare these boys and girls with "normals," control children who were the same age were selected by teachers at school or from the neighborhood (if the visit was to the home), and they were given the same battery of psychological tests as the subjects.

Haraldsson's team expressed their appreciation, after the testing, with gifts of sweets and ballpoint pens to the children, and found all the families to be cooperative and helpful. Sri Lanka (formerly Ceylon) is predominantly Buddhist, and while this belief system differs from that of the Hindu, it does allow for rebirth.

So, how did the comparison turn out? Relative to a control sample, children claiming previous-life memories were actually smarter, had better memory skills, and were doing much better in school than their peers. They also tended to be more serious in their studies, clowning around less, and were perfectionists. Although a bit more argumentative and stubborn, they were not socially isolated. Their test scores did not show them to be particularly suggestible.

It is Haraldsson's impression that these children are sincerely convinced as to the reality of their alleged memories, and that simple déjà vu (a common phenomenon that affects all age groups, is transient, and lacks coherency and detail) does not explain them.

Gory Details

As if the foregoing were not disquieting enough, there is another aspect of Stevenson's work that is, for lack of a more scientific term, creepy. Consider the case of Corliss Chotkin, Jr.,[12] a Native American of Tlingit lineage in southeastern Alaska. The Tlingits have a belief in reincarnation that predates contact with European culture and persists to this day, although mostly in the elder generation.

The Tlingits' take on this is that most "returns" are intrafamilial, may be foretold by the dying person, and can be verified by birthmarks. An elderly, dying Tlingit named Victor Vincent told a favorite niece, Irene Chotkin, that he would be reborn as her son. To press his point, and to make sure that Irene would recognize his arrival, he showed her two scars — one on his nose and one on his back — from past minor surgeries. The back scar had the signature look of a sewn-up wound: little stitch-hole scars straddling it.

Victor died in 1946. Irene gave birth to Corliss Jr. (named after his father) eighteen months later. Stevenson investigated the case during a series of visits in the early 1960s. He found the usual declamation by the toddler, in this case at thirteen months, that he was "Kahkody," Victor Vincent's tribal name. In later

12 ibid.

years, Corliss also recognized people whom Victor had known (people Corliss had never previously met). Corliss spoke about events in Victor's life about which he had no knowledge; he combed his hair and even stuttered just like the old man.

Then there were also the birthmarks. Corliss Jr. was born with two—in exactly the same spots where Victor Vincent had pointed them out on his own body. When Stevenson examined him, Corliss was already a teenager and had lost his stutter and his memories of being Kahkody, but the birthmark on the back was a thick line over an inch long, with dots on each side, surgical-suture style.

Stevenson finds birthmarks or birth defects in over a third of his cases. And these almost invariably correspond to wounds or existing marks on the previous personality. Thus, if the original person was shot in the abdomen and killed, the baby who will claim to be this victim may have a pair of birthmarks, one front, one back, as if in remembrance of the bullet's entrance and exit.

Susan Eastland had a birthmark (medically, a nevus) on her left hip. When Stevenson obtained a copy of Winnie Eastland's medical records, the point of impact of the car that struck and killed her was at this very spot.

Another piece of this bizarre puzzle has to do with dreams. The Eastlands' older daughter had a dream, six months after Winnie's death, that Winnie would return to the family. When Charlotte Eastland became pregnant two years later, the daughter again had such a dream. Now, dreams are often wish fulfillments, and one can see why a grieving sister might dream this way. Dreams often have a way of being remembered if something in them ultimately rings true, and forgotten when they seem irrelevant. Yet Stevenson finds a similar pattern—of pertinent dreams preceding the birth of a child who will claim to be someone else—often enough to consider this an occasional part of the package. As previously noted, we don't know why we bother to dream anyway. . . .

Stevenson's "classical" case (he uses the term "fully developed case") contains five features: a prediction of rebirth, a dream, a birthmark or defect, statements by the child about the previous life, and associated unusual behavior. Of course, as is usually the situation in medicine, individual cases are rarely fully classical. Stevenson rarely finds all five items together. While the core features of cases are the same worldwide, some of the variations occur within cultures.

Reincarnation Around the World

For about forty years, beginning in 1960, Ian Stevenson traveled the world researching these unusual children. While all cultures harbor some, there are certain areas, usually where the people accept reincarnation, in which the cases are found more easily. These include northern India, Sri Lanka, Myanmar, Thailand, parts of Turkey, Lebanon (among the Druse), Syria, West Africa, and the Tlingits of Alaska. It is not surprising that cultures that subscribe to reincarnation produce more cases, as a child is more likely to be taken seriously in these venues. But Stevenson also finds cases in Europe and North America, where the belief is minimal, and notes frequent suppression of cases in areas where it's accepted, because of fear, jealousy, or inconvenience. For case-finding, Stevenson relies on associates and other people he's worked with (e.g., interpreters) in foreign countries, and on calls and letters from Americans who've seen something about his work in the media. Basically, once he started researching cases, he had no trouble finding them.

Reincarnation-friendly societies vary in their beliefs and manifestations. The Tlingits feel that one can specify the family into which they will re-emerge. (This was true in the case presented above; Stevenson found this tidbit in ten of the forty-six Tlingit cases he studied.) Heraldic dreams are common in Myanmar, and occur before conception; they are also common among the Tlingits, but tend to occur in the last month of the pregnancy. Same-family returns constitute most of the solved cases in Myanmar, Thailand, Nigeria (among the Igbo), and the lower forty-eight U.S. states, but are rare in India and Sri Lanka. Opposite-sex redux varies from zero to 50 percent, by area (it's 15 percent in the U.S.).

Despite these variations, the essential features—the onset at about age three, the stubborn persistence of the child as to who he or she really is, the rapid and near-complete disappearance of the syndrome at about age seven—are fairly consistent globally. The time interval from death to reappearance varies, but the median is relatively short—about fifteen months. Reportage rates vary greatly, and the majority of cases likely go unreported. Still, this condition is rare. Most children, in fact, do not espouse a prior life. Those that do are aberrations, and some twist of nature is perhaps responsible.

Why Am I Like This?

In medicine, many diseases exist in subclinical forms. Symptoms may be mild or nonexistent, but laboratory testing shows the disease to have occurred. For the West Nile virus, for example, over a hundred people become infected for each one who actually gets sick. Mononucleosis and hepatitis, particularly in children, are usually asymptomatic.

Consequently, Stevenson wonders if there are lesser, incomplete forms of the previous-life phenomenon, such as a strong personality trait or penchant appearing in a child within a family where it would be unusual. Corliss Chotkin, Jr. had a fascination with engines, and a precocious ability to operate and repair them. He didn't learn this from his father, who was far from mechanically inclined. But Victor Vincent had repaired engines. Stevenson cites another case of a boy who had a fascination with watches, as well as an uncanny ability to repair them, in a family where watchmaking was quite alien.

Further conjecture along these lines includes the differences between identical twins. With precisely the same genetic material, twins arising from a single sperm–egg union (known as monozygotic), even when raised together and in the same way, often show differences. A new branch of science called epigenetics tries to explain this by showing how some genes can be activated or de-activated so that the same DNA may drive a cell in different directions. A newspaper report about this research refers to the process as "a mysterious biological mechanism." Which is to say, even if we know *how* the body steers a cell in a particular direction, we still don't know *why*.

Among the University of Virginia's twenty-five hundred reincarnation-type cases are forty-two identical-twin pairs where *both* twins had memories of previous lives. Thirty-one of these are solved: Two previously living persons (each corresponding to one twin's memories) were identified. These "corresponding pairs," interestingly, had usually been related to each other, like husband and wife. Needless to say, these twins' personality differences and relationships to each other resembled those of their earlier counterparts, however their genes lined up to express this.

Then there are the children whose current sex differs from their "previous" one. Cross-dressing and other gender-inappropriate behavior may be seen. Stevenson followed some of these children into adulthood, and found that most had come to accept their bodies and their genders. I suspect that in the times and cultures in which this happened, "coming out" was, shall we say, less fashionable than it currently is in the U.S., and same-sex orientation may have been more frequent than it appeared. Stevenson considers homosexuality a possible outcome of male/female reincarnative mismatch. As I noted in chapter 6, no one else as yet has come up with a better explanation.

Process and Outcome

Whatever process Stevenson has spent his life studying, he stops short of labeling it "reincarnation." An earlier book (1974) was titled *20 Cases Suggestive of Reincarnation*. The most recent work (2001), which I cited at this chapter's beginning is subtitled *A Question of Reincarnation*. At other times, Stevenson has referred to "cases of the *reincarnation-type*" (all emphasis mine).

In the 2001 book, he reflects about some other implications. He is often asked about the math: Since more people are alive today than at any previous time, from whence do their spirits derive? Aside from the fact that the number of all the people who ever walked this planet is greater than the earth's current population, or that souls might be created as needed, he replies that a reincarnation need not be one-to-one, or that multiple bodies might share one mind (as the Igbo of Nigeria and the Inuit believe), or that animals may at times occupy positions in the cycle of birth/rebirth (as the Hindus and Buddhists believe).

As to the preponderance of violent deaths among the cases, are these simply more memorable? Or might such avenues of dying focus the karma more sharply? Why do children, if they remember at all, only remember one life? Is it because that is the one most recent? Why do genetics and environment, the scientific one-two punch of all biologic determinism, fail to explain many personality traits and illnesses?

What about individuals who, as children, seemed to "know" their destinies? Stevenson cites Florence Nightingale, who as a small child doctored her dolls and ultimately went into nursing despite her parents' objections. St. Catherine of Siena fasted and scourged herself and played hermit in her early childhood. Although her parents were pious, nothing in their lives presaged their daughter's path to sainthood. While these examples, unlike Stevenson's "typical case," never morphed away from their childhood personae nor specified a findable person who they claimed to be, one wonders how a child so clearly sees a road that no one else can see.

Of course, we only notice the ones whose paths lead to fame. In my contemporary culture, Bob Dylan imagined himself, early on, as an archetypal American Folksinger. While his mother's family owned theaters, I have never heard mention of any of his relatives being a serious performer or musician. Although some considered his act phony in that it belied his middle-class Jewish upbringing, a sense of self is not a simple thing to trace. In a *60 Minutes* interview (December 5, 2004), Dylan told Ed Bradley that he knew as a boy that he was destined to become a music legend. He said he changed his name (from Robert Allen Zimmerman) because "you're born, you know, the wrong names, wrong parents." He said he had no idea how he wrote his great songs of the sixties, that they were "almost magically written." In a PBS broadcast (September 26, 2005), *No Direction Home*, Dylan reiterated: "I was born very far from where I'm supposed to be . . ." and ". . . not even born to the right parents or something. . . ."

Another example: the Reverend Al Sharpton. According to a *New Yorker* profile (February 18, 2002), he began preaching "almost as soon" as he could talk. He would regularly arrange his sister's dolls as a congregation, don his mother's bathrobe, and preach using a candle as a microphone. In public school, he would only sign his name as "Reverend Alfred Sharpton." No one knew where this came from, and no one could make him stop doing it. (He did ultimately accept advice to shorten "Alfred" to "Al".)

How does a four-year-old have a sense of destiny? How does a child claim to really be someone else, and supply verifiable details of the life of another person that he could not possibly have known? Stevenson ruled out fraud in all but a very few cases. He also ruled out a forgotten source of the information, because there are too many families where this would have been impossible. How is the information acquired? Telepathy? Possession? Stevenson considers these, but favors some sort of survival of personality after death.

I have no explanation either, but the findings and the thorough, meticulous research of the cases that has been Stevenson's life work are undeniable. Reviewing one of his earlier works, in 1975, the *Journal of the American Medical Association* notes that while he may not convince skeptics, he has "painstakingly and unemotionally . . . placed on record a large amount of data that cannot be ignored." Read one of his books and see for yourself.

Part 2

$\int$ixteen

One Person's Paranormal Is Another Person's Science: Acupuncture

An American ear, nose, and throat surgeon from New York's Mount Sinai Hospital traveled to China in 1971, when the first trickle of Westerners was being allowed to do so. Dr. Samuel Rosen was invited to show the Chinese an operation to restore hearing that he had developed, and to witness Chinese medicine. One thing he witnessed was something he couldn't have imagined; this description is taken from his autobiography.

A Most Unusual Scenario
The patient was a forty-year-old man, a physician himself, suffering from tuberculosis that could not be eradicated with drugs. He needed part of his lung removed—a lobe infested with the germs—to cure, or at least control, his disease. A lobe

is a sizeable piece of lung, up to a third, and getting to it requires what is known in medical slang as "cracking the chest."

This, unfortunately, is very much like it sounds; but if you're a surgeon doing it every day, you develop a businesslike detachment: You might as well be cracking an egg. Needless to say, this operation requires anesthesia well beyond what a few shots of novocaine can do, because thoracotomy (the non-slang term) necessitates breaking ribs.

In what he describes as a familiar, standard operating room, Dr. Rosen watched the anesthesiologist—an acupuncturist—clean the patient's right forearm with alcohol, select a fine, stainless-steel needle, and then insert it, almost an inch deep, into the outer forearm about halfway between the wrist and elbow. Keep in mind that in 1971, almost no one in the U.S. had ever heard of acupuncture, let alone seen it, so this doctor from New York was already bewildered.

The Chinese practitioner began to twirl the needle; she continued this for about twenty minutes, occasionally questioning the patient about his sensations. She nodded to the surgeon, and then Dr. Rosen saw something he couldn't believe. Without hesitating, the surgeon sliced an incision over a foot long from back around to front, while the American braced himself for the patient's screams. They never came. Which was good, because then it was time to crack the chest. With a scissors-like instrument, the surgeon began cutting ribs, in their entirety, away from the breastbone, so they could then be spread, opening a window in which the heart and lungs could be seen.

All this while the patient was awake. He sipped some tea as the nurse held the teakettle spout to his lips. He conversed with the surgeon, who showed him the removed section of lung for a quick medical consultation as to whether this looked adequate. It did.

The surgeon closed. The patient, smiling and comfortable, sat up and bade his "American friends" goodbye, and was wheeled away.

All told, Samuel Rosen watched fifteen major surgeries under acupuncture anesthesia, including operations on the brain, stomach, thyroid, and tonsils. As strange as this appeared to a Westerner, it worked.

James Reston Visits China

That same year, *New York Times* columnist James Reston traveled to China, where he ended up needing an emergency appendectomy. Although a more conventional type of anesthesia was used for the operation itself, on the second night afterward, Mr. Reston had a lot of abdominal pain. Rather than a shot of morphine, an acupuncturist was called in, with Reston's approval. Long, thin needles were inserted into the outer right elbow and below the knees, and these were manipulated to enhance the effect. Reston at first thought this a rather complicated—not to mention circuitous—way of dealing with his pain, as the needles were inserted at locations far from the pain itself.

But . . . an hour later, the pain and the abdominal gas distention abated and did not return. Reston was struck by the unusual nature of the treatment he had received and, being a columnist, wrote about it ("Now, let me tell you about my appendectomy in Peking . . . ," *New York Times,* July 26, 1971). This was the first mass-media introduction to acupuncture in the United States.

A Blast From the Past

The history of acupuncture goes back several thousand years, overlapping Judeo-Christian biblical times. Its origins are a little obscure, but most historians cite a basis within the philosophy of Chinese medicine having to do with energy flows through the body and a need to balance them. It was not used exclusively by the Chinese; a system sounding like acupuncture was described in an Egyptian papyrus, and forms of healing based on stimulation of far-away points can be found in a variety of cultures. When a frozen five-thousand-year-old man was found in a glacier way up in the Alps of northern Italy in 1991, his unusually well-preserved body showed, some believe, tattoo evidence of acupuncture treatment.

Other tales of its provenance are more practically and empirically based. Ancient warriors who had been shot with arrows in certain areas of the body couldn't help but notice that chronic ailments elsewhere got better as a result. Or huddled around a fire in olden times, flying embers accidentally burned specific body areas, resulting—lo and behold—in an unexpected cure of something. (Acupuncture points, in fact, don't have to be needled —they can be lightly burned as well. The herb moxa [mugwort] is used for this, and the process is known as moxibustion.)

However it developed, acupuncture, upon its arrival in the West, appeared sufficiently strange to be considered . . . paranormal. In fact, a symposium on the topic at Stanford University in 1972 was sponsored by a California organization known as the Academy of Parapsychology and Medicine. The program was hosted not by the Stanford Medical School, which thought it too weird, but by the Department of Industrial Engineering and Materials Science. Fourteen hundred physicians attended (twice the number expected).

This information derives from a paper in the *Journal of the American Medical Women's Association* later that year, by Stanford psychiatrist J. Elizabeth Jeffress, who entitled the piece

"Acupuncture: Witchcraft or Wizardry?". She concluded "that the failure to understand how it works should not deter us from using acupuncture."

Acceptance of the Craft

In my professional lifetime, acupuncture has moved over a long bridge. It is now practically mainstream. Insurance often pays for it. Veterinarians use it on animals. Our National Institutes of Health (NIH), in a 1998 consensus statement, found "promising results" in the treatment of dental pain and of the nausea and vomiting that follow chemotherapy or surgery. "May be useful" was the designation for a host of other conditions. The point, as it were, is that acupuncture's effectiveness has been validated via scientific study for a variety of conditions.

Here's an example, from the *Journal of the American Medical Association (JAMA)*, in the November 11, 1998 issue: "Moxibustion for Correction of Breech Presentation, a Randomized Controlled Trial." Breech presentation is when a baby comes out bottom first, and it's a difficult delivery (in this country, it usually means a Caesarian section). The infant's position in the womb can be ascertained by ultrasound images, so it needn't be a delivery-room surprise.

Breech orientation in the womb is common early in a pregnancy, but the small, mobile fetus often rights itself into the correct position. Attempts can be made to manipulate it into alignment by pushing from the outside. Sometimes this works, but there is another way: moxibustion. As mentioned, this is the burning of moxa at specific locations corresponding to acupuncture points.

The study was done in China. The 130 women studied were thirty-three weeks pregnant with their first child. All had ultrasound-confirmed breech-positioned fetuses. The 130 were "randomized": Half got the usual prenatal care; the other half got that, plus moxibustion. This meant firing up a cigar-shaped roll of moxa and singeing, as much as the patient could stand, the outside of each little toe. This is the location of a particular acupoint; it was cooked, you could say, until it was red and short of blistering, fifteen minutes on each fifth toe. That's thirty minutes a day, and daily treatment was given for a week. If baby hadn't turned by then, another week of therapy was given.

After two weeks, the trial stopped, and any pregnancy still a breech was referred for the standard turning procedure. It is hard to have control patients in an acupuncture study, since it's a little obvious who's getting the real McCoy. You can stimulate areas that aren't known acupoints, but sometimes even that has a therapeutic effect. In the treated group, three-quarters of the fetuses converted to a normal (vertex) lie; in the usual care ("control") group, slightly less than half corrected. Increased fetal motion was noted in the treatment group; presumably this enabled the redirection.

In other words, burning a little mugwort on the outsides of your pinky toes rights your fetus's position. I read it in the *Journal of the American Medical Association*. And if I had read it somewhere else, and if it had been called witchcraft, I wouldn't have known the difference.

In fact, in 1995, Japanese acupuncturist and physician Yoshiaki Omura went to Brazil and observed several psychic healers. Omura had been one of the first acupuncturists to demonstrate acupuncture anesthesia in the United States in the early 1970s. The healing ritual he watched in Sao Paulo included sham surgery, some real minor surgery, and injection of a strange-looking liquid. Omura noted that the injections were at known acupuncture points, and that the healer twirled the needle, as an acupuncturist would. Other aspects of the process also looked familiar. Pointing fingers at patients without touching them resembled a Qi Gong distant-healing technique. Massage and a manual procedure appeared to be a form of chiropractic manipulation. In other words, what looked like a primitive healing ritual actually contained aspects of known medical processes. Omura's "Impression of Observing Psychic Surgery and Healing in Brazil Which Appear to Incorporate Qi Gong Energy and the Use of Acupuncture Points" was published in *Acupuct Electrother Research* in 1997.

Uses

What are the therapeutic uses of acupuncture? As seen in the opening example, it can be used for surgical anesthesia. I remember a brief time, after acupuncture first made its way westward, when people wondered if it would replace our standard inhalation anesthesia, colloquially known as "gas." It seemed as though American anesthesiologists risked obsolescence.

This never happened. Aside from all the politics that would have been involved, gas is basically a sure thing. You may have to give a little more sometimes, and there is always the risk of a serious allergic reaction, but your patient won't start kicking on the operating table while your hands are inside his abdomen. Acupuncture, for whatever reason, doesn't work on everyone, and may work better for some areas of the body than others. I understand that in China nowadays, most surgical anesthesia is done as we do it here, and sometimes for a very American reason: the reimbursement is better!

It is for pain relief that acupuncture is perhaps best known. The NIH consensus report (which had been published in *JAMA*) cited its demonstrated ability to relieve post-operative dental pain. There were "reasonable studies" that it was effective for menstrual cramps, tennis elbow, and fibromyalgia. More recent studies show acupuncture to be efficacious for osteoarthritis of the knee. This is the most common type of knee arthritis, particularly in older people, and this 2004 study in the *Annals of Internal Medicine* enrolled 570 patients. The three treatment groups got true acupuncture, "sham" acupuncture (the needles didn't actually puncture the skin, but were taped to it), or group-education sessions. True treatment reduced pain by 40 percent, which was greater than the results in the other two categories, although the "sham" subjects did better than the education group.

The results of a single study are often promising but need independent confirmation. The *Annals* published a 2005 analysis of twenty-two trials of acupuncture for chronic low-back pain. Needling was more effective than doing nothing, but only comparable at best to massage or medication, and not as good as spinal manipulation.

Two studies of acupuncture for headache demonstrate another problem. A study of 401 patients in England, in the *British Medical Journal (BMJ)*, compared twelve acupuncture treatments over three months with "usual care." It concluded: "Acupuncture leads to persisting, clinically relevant benefits for primary care patients with chronic headache, particularly migraine. Expansion of National Health Service acupuncture services should be considered." A 2005 paper in *JAMA* comparing twelve sessions (over eight weeks) of true, sham, or no

acupuncture found real and sham acupuncture equally effective
and better than no treatment. Sham therapy in this case was the
needling of non-acupuncture points.

This highlights a recurrent problem in evaluating acupuncture studies. Since the "placebo effect" of any medical intervention is improvement, at least temporarily, in about 40
percent of patients, any proof of a treatment's effectiveness
must use a comparison group of people who only *believe* they
were treated. This is easy enough with pills: the placebos only
need to look like the real thing. But subjects know whether or
not they're being stuck with pins. True acupuncture uses
known, specific points where needles are applied for particular
conditions. Sham treatment may use other points. Surpris-
ingly, such "pretend" treatment sometimes appears effective,
as in the *JAMA* headache study above. The *JAMA* authors conclude, as if unimpressed, that "Acupuncture was no more
effective than sham acupuncture in reducing migraine
headaches," but remark that both fared better than no needles
at all. The British study, where the control group simply got
their usual medical care and nobody got simulated acupuncture, is more enthusiastic. Even though both studies note that
treatment helps, acupuncture is found no better than placebo
by *JAMA* and worthy of government investment by the *BMJ*.

A 2000 *JAMA* paper looked at women with breast cancer
receiving chemotherapy, to see if acupuncture could reduce the
associated nausea and vomiting. This time electroacupuncture
was used; this means the needles were connected via alligator
clips to a battery (some believe this enhances the effect).
Control patients were lightly needled at non-points and the battery, although connected, was not turned on. A third group got
neither of the above. Electroacupuncture was clearly better than

mock therapy, and mock treatment was better than nothing at all. This is more in line with what researchers hope to achieve: There is a real and measurable effect of just believing one has been treated, but the response to true therapy is better than placebo.

Acupuncture has an interesting history in treating addictions. Some of medicine's best discoveries (like penicillin) have been accidental. In 1972, Dr. H. L. Wen, a Hong Kong neurosurgeon, was in the process of anesthetizing a patient who happened to be an opium addict, and when a needle was applied to the ear, the patient unexpectedly announced that he had lost his craving for opium. British surgeon Dr. Margaret Patterson was training in Hong Kong at the time; she learned about the technique and brought it back to England, with a few refinements. Her patients did well with it, as did the cocaine-addicted patients of Dr. Michael Smith at Lincoln Hospital in the Bronx, New York, but randomized, controlled trials — considered a research gold standard — have mostly failed to demonstrate a benefit.

Acupuncture vs. Hypnosis

Unlike hypnosis, acupuncture has been unsuccessful in published trials for alleviating irritable bowel syndrome. Also, there are no significant papers to suggest that it will rid you of warts (as hypnosis might). Yet it is tempting to make some comparisons. Both have been used since time immemorial; both can provide surgical anesthesia and pain relief, and can lessen chemotherapy-associated vomiting. Both are hard to study by comparison to "control" subjects. And both require considerable practitioner skill along with amenable patients. Acupuncture can be used on animals, who presumably don't bend to the power of hypnotic suggestion. Human fetuses are also not presumed to be suggestible, but a 1994 study in the *Archives of Family Medicine* achieved conversion of breech to normal delivery position in about the same proportions of women as in the moxibustion paper, above, only they used hypnosis.

Acupuncture versus hypnosis was tested in a 1997 study on male sexual dysfunction in Istanbul, Turkey. Sexual function improved by about 45 percent with placebo (as would be expected), 60 percent with acupuncture, and 75 percent with hypnosis. The numbers of patients treated were insufficient, however, to reach statistical significance. In a 2001 comparison at the University of Pennsylvania's dental school, patients with head and neck pain were studied. Acute (recent onset) pain benefited most from acupuncture, while those with psychogenic pain (having a psychological rather than a physiological origin) did better with hypnosis. In "Mechanism of Analgesia Induced by Hypnosis and Acupuncture: Is There a Difference?" in the journal *Pain* in 1991, a Swiss team, using volunteers who immersed their hands in ice water until it hurt, found that acupuncture and hypnosis both significantly reduced the pain, but that neither seemed to work through the body's natural opiate (endorphin) system.

How It Works

The bulk of the evidence, however, seems to favor an endorphin link to acupuncture's effect. Much of this work has been done in animals. An experiment on rabbits in the 1970s showed that the fluid that bathes the brain and spinal cord taken from one rabbit following acupuncture and then injected into a second rabbit appeared to confer pain relief; something in the fluid was transferable.

In other studies, the drug naloxone, which blocks the effects of opiate (i.e., narcotic) pain killers, also blocks the pain-diminishing quality of acupuncture. It was discovered in the 1970s that our brains contain receptor sites for opiates, as if these narcotic-type drugs serve some physiologic purpose. Since everything the body does must ultimately make sense, soon afterward came the discovery that the body makes opiates, which we call endorphins, to bind to these sites, providing in a natural way what painkillers accomplish.

Acupuncture, and particularly electroacupuncture, where an electric current is applied to the needle, have been shown to increase the body's production of these endorphins, particularly at certain currents. This could explain why pain is relieved. Other explanations propose that the pin-sticking sensation may jam other pain signals to produce anesthesia. Although this sounds a little like telling someone to pinch their thigh real hard so as not to notice that they have a toothache, the purported mechanism is more complex.

The Chinese view acupuncture as a way to manipulate the flow of energy (which they call "Qi") through channels they know as meridians. These meridians, twelve in all, are elusive when searched for by Western scientific techniques. But the acupuncture points themselves can be demonstrated electrically. An American team consisting of two biophysicists and an orthopedist published "Electrical Correlates of Acupuncture Points" in a MEDLINE-indexed electrical engineering journal in 1975.

They showed that many of the centuries-old traditional Chinese acupuncture points could be found electrically, and in the same spots in different patients. These tiny areas had a slightly positive charge relative to surrounding tissue. They conducted electricity better, which is to say that their electrical resistance was lower. This fact is the basis for gadgets sold as acupuncture-point finders. While a metal plate touches the skin elsewhere, a metal probe slides around the skin searching for points. Encountering one, a circuit is completed through the body via the plate, causing a buzzer in the device to sound or a bulb to light. No self-respecting acupuncturist would use one of these things (why would they *need* to, anyway?), and readings can be thrown off by moisture on the skin or how hard you push the probe, but I've played around with an inexpensive point finder (prices now begin at about $150), and I can tell you that the same points buzz/light consistently, whether I slide it over my own hand or my cat's ear. Acupuncture points are real; you can't find them with a microscope, but proper electrical equipment does the trick.

It is not clear why needling of non-points, in controlled, clinical studies, sometimes produces the same effect as true point treatment. Some trials with electroacupuncture show endorphin release that's independent of where the stimulus is placed. Psychiatry professor George Ulett of the University of Missouri, writing in the *Skeptical Inquirer* (2003), feels acupuncture to be "a potent technique giving lasting relief from chronic pain." Endorphin release explains its effects, he says, not a metaphysical system of meridians and Qi.

Endorphins, as I mentioned, were discovered during the 1970s. Does that mean that acupuncture was witchcraft in 1970 and science in 1980? Much of what is in this book simply awaits the scientific discoveries that will pull it from paranormal/metaphysical into mainstream respectability. Remember that in 1972, Stanford University's medical school wouldn't host an acupuncture conference. Now, even a skeptic realizes that the technique works, and offers a scientific explanation. Progress.

When I first read Dr. Rosen's report of how one pin stuck and twirled in the forearm allowed a chest to be cracked open, I wondered if there was an organ system in the body that had not been discovered. Perhaps this system had to do with the flow of electricity through the body and its resultant effects on the body's chemistry. Acupuncture anesthesia may be accomplished through endorphin release, but you cannot give someone enough morphine to operate on them while they're still conscious. Nerve signal interference doesn't quite seem to explain how a man comfortably takes a few sips of tea while there's a gaping hole in his chest. And why would stimulation of certain parts of the skin trigger endorphin release in the brain, anyway? Why does the stimulation have to be done in a specific way, whether it's by applying an electric current (only certain currents work) or twirling a needle? We don't know, but we're getting there. Acupuncture is respectable now, and its mechanisms are at least partially understood.

Seventeen
Life as a Hologram

Karl Lashley, mentioned earlier, ended his quest for the physical mechanisms of memory in frustration, as he could not localize storage sites. In 1946, a young neurosurgeon named Karl Pribram came to work with him.

The Hologram is Born

One year later, the Hungarian physicist Dennis Gabor was looking for a way to get better resolution through an electron microscope. He used a form of calculus (devised by the Frenchman Jean B. J. Fourier in the eighteenth century) that showed how any pattern could be translated into waveforms, which could then be converted back to the original pattern. Using light beams, made of waves, he produced the first—albeit crude—holograms. Since each light wave used bounced off the object and then spread onto the entire surface of the film, each point on the film contained information sufficient to reconstruct the whole object. More points merely meant better clarity. Impressed by this, Gabor christened the image a hologram, Greek for the "whole message." He would later win a Nobel Prize for it.

When lasers came along in 1960, their unique light was ideal for producing holograms, and these are the sort you see today. They are formed when two laser beams coming from the same source intersect, one coming off the object to be "photographed," the other acting as a reference. The resulting interference pattern contains the information needed to reconstruct the image. This is a difficult concept for most of us to grasp (I don't fully understand it either), but the three-dimensional holograms that ensue can be stunning. Some holographic images are projected in such a way as to allow us to walk around them, full circle, seeing the object as it would look from all sides.

Holographic Memory

Karl Pribram became fascinated by memory's anatomic mystery and by the fact that removing sizeable chunks of brain tissue only made it fuzzier without obliterating anything, just like in a hologram. But Pribram carried this past the metaphor stage. In his book *Languages of the Brain* (1971), he theorized that neural activity and perception produce hologram-like interference patterns within the brain. These patterns could serve as the basis for memories that behave as if they were somehow distributed through large parts of the brain. Dr. Pribram, currently a Distinguished Research Professor at Georgetown University, has recently embellished his theory with some mathematics and quantum physics.

The fact that holograms can be reconstructed from any part of the picture is also a feature of memory. Since different areas of the brain process, for example, vision, hearing, smell, or emotion, it has never been quite understood how any part of a memory can bring up all the parts. A rose — red, fragrant, thorny, beautiful, perhaps associated with sunshine or being outdoors — flashes into memory in its entirety, even though the memory is evoked by only one of its components (like seeing something red). Holographic patterning within the brain would explain this. In Pribram's words, "What better mechanism can be operating than the associative recall provided by the holographic process?"

Holograms also have the ability to store huge amounts of easily retrievable information in tiny spaces — as does the brain. Although the movement of molecules within the nervous system generates electrical activity, including waves, Pribram notes that holography does not necessarily depend on waves. He cites a computer program that uses Fourier's mathematics, upon which holography is based, that constructs holograms that are not based on light.

Pribram goes on to describe experiments on human vision that show a relationship with Fourier holograms. He believes that the junctions between nerve cells (synapses) generate small electrical waves, in addition to simply passing an impulse from one nerve fiber to the next. The interaction, or superposition, of these waves would behave holographically, and in accordance with Fourier's mathematics.

This Looks Familiar

Now let's mention déjà vu. Again. Literally it means "already seen." This phenomenon of suddenly having a feeling of familiarity, like you've been there before, can be found in 30 to 96 percent of the population, depending on the study. Most of these feelings qualify as normal—just another aspect of the human experience. Occasionally, in the context of an ongoing mental illness, they can be prolonged, frightening, and reality-bending. An interesting article in *The American Journal of Psychiatry* in 1990 is appropriate here.

In "The Déjà Vu Experience: Remembrance of Things Past?", two Dutch psychiatrists take a comprehensive look at the process. Common as it is, the cause is generally not clear. In rare cases, electrical activity in the brain's temporal lobes, which are intimately associated with memory, triggers déjà vu. Wilder Penfield, the neurosurgeon (described earlier) who evoked memories by electrical stimulation of the temporal lobes as he searched for the source area of a patient's epilepsy, was able to find a spot that reproduced a sense of déjà vu in six of 214 patients. In some patients, a temporal lobe-based seizure disorder manifests only with recurrent, strong déjà vu sensations. This is unusual, but it has been known to happen. Why activation of a particular brain area would elicit a sense of having "been there before" is another story.

The authors review all the published speculations as to why most of us occasionally feel like we've seen it all before. Anxiety. Exhaustion. Emotional trauma. Stress. Fatigue. Drugs. None of these does it justice, as most déjà vu is just . . . normal. Paranormal explanations would include intrusions from past lives, telepathy, or recall of things seen during an out-of-body episode. These don't settle the issue either. Freud wrote that déjà vu could be the result of a dream, or could even occur during a dream. Enter holography.

The article ends with a discussion of technological models. The authors believe that holograms would explain how a complete memory is reconstructed by stimulating only one section of the brain, and why a memory fails to disappear if this section is removed. They speculate that an indistinct, out-of-focus fragment of a holographic memory might match an entering image as it begins to form in memory. The result: a brief sense of recognition.

Oh . . . the Pain

In the journal *Geriatrics* (2002), Dr. Albert L. Ray, medical director of the Miami Pain and Integrative Medicine Center, talks about the pain hologram. Here, the term is metaphoric: Pain is a complex interaction of input signals from the damaged area, a localization process so you know just where you hurt, an emotional reaction based on your baseline level of inner peace and a remembrance of pains past. Ray calls it "a projection of multiple components that come together." Holograms, as mentioned, are formed by projections of interacting rays of light. Ray gives examples of older patients with neck and shoulder pain from spinal disc disease; fear or ongoing stress turns up the volume; another patient with the same disc herniation feels no pain at all.

The Holographic Universe

But wait, there's more. Jacob D. Bekenstein, professor of theoretical physics and laureate of the Israel Prize in physics in 2005, wrote an article for *Scientific American* (August 2003). With the title "Information in the Holographic Universe," this astrophysicist likens our universe to one giant hologram.

A hologram is created when two just-so beams of light intersect. This interference pattern is captured on what is essentially a high-resolution photographic film. The picture recorded is incomprehensible, looking like TV "snow"—until you shine laser light through it. Then the entire image is reconstructed, projected into space in three dimensions. Bekenstein's point is that the flat, two-dimensional film codes the information for a 3-D reality. He believes that this 2-D encoding explains the physics of space's black holes—regions so dense that their gravity sucks in everything around them, even light. He cites data showing that whatever we can learn about a region of space is defined by its (2-D) surface area, not its (3-D) volume. He hopes this finding "is a clue to the ultimate theory of reality."

The increasing sophistication of biology and chemistry has resulted in a what-you-see-is-what-you-get attitude toward life. Acupuncture works by releasing endorphin molecules; low brain oxygen causes near-death perceptions. Everything is explainable at a molecular level. It all fits together like an erector set. Biochemistry has given us amazing advances in medicine and physiology; we've mapped the entire human genome. But there are enough things that we don't fully understand to enlist mathematics and physics as well. Karl Pribram believes that some brain processes are best understood by "coordinated mathematics." Waveforms carry detailed information (think television). There is no reason to have to understand all that we observe using only existing principles. Science will march on.

$\mathcal{E}$ighteen

The Orthopedist and the Body Electric: Life's Electromagnetic Template

Robert O. Becker, M.D., now retired and in his eighties, was a professor of orthopedic surgery at the Upstate Medical Center in Syracuse, New York. He has long been interested in how electricity and magnetism, in minute amounts—nothing you could feel or sense—might affect bodily function.

Of Tomatoes, Salamanders, and Frogs

In 1957, the Russians launched Sputnik, the first satellite. This took the American government somewhat by surprise, as the Russians were believed to have insufficient technology to do this. Hurriedly, the government started translating Soviet scientific journals into English and distributing them to federally funded institutions, like Veterans' Administration hospitals. Dr. Becker was working at the VA Medical Center in

Syracuse at the time, and the library received a crate of Russian journals every month; he seemed to be the only one interested.

It was obvious from the journals that the Russians were willing to pursue and fund research that would be considered outlandish and unworthy here. What's more, if the research turned up something unexpected or unexplainable, they were willing to publish it. In the U.S., if you don't get the expected result, it's not so easy to get your work into print.

An item in a biophysics journal caught Becker's eye. It had to do with tiny amounts of naturally occurring electricity within plants. Cutting branches off tomato plants, the Russian author was able to measure an electrical "current of injury" at the stumps, which seemed to help the plants regrow the lost part. This current changed direction over time, and could be manipulated with small batteries, so that with just the right flow, the plant could regenerate up to three times faster, or not at all!

Two centuries earlier, an Italian priest named Lazzaro Spallanzini had discovered that adult salamanders could regenerate many parts of their bodies: legs, tail, even a jaw. It was well known that plants could re-form lopped-off pieces, but an animal with four legs and eyes? This was something else. Twenty years earlier, a young naturalist from Geneva had found a quarter-inch-long pond creature that could grow back its entire head or body and named it the hydra, after the mythical beast that could accomplish the same.

Subsequently, Luigi Galvani, a Bolognese anatomy professor, demonstrated that an electrical current developed in the wounds of severed frogs' legs. The invention, about thirty years later, of the galvanometer (named after him), which

measures electrical current, made this injury-generated phenomenon easier to observe. Over time came the discoveries
that nerve impulses travel electrically, although not as they do
in a wire, and that the communication between nerve cells happens through released chemical "transmitters." This latter discovery was made by Otto Loewi at the NYU School of
Medicine. He won a Nobel Prize for it in 1936. The idea sup-
posedly came to him in a dream. He awoke realizing he'd had
the dream but could not remember it; the next night, he had the
same dream, remembered it, and did the definitive experiment
the next day.

Of Stem Cells and Broken Bones

Becker began doing research on the salamander and its cells; he
noticed that strange things could happen to the red blood cells
around a current of injury. Within the blood clot that formed to
stanch the bleeding, some of the cells slowly changed: They
became what would now be called stem cells. But then, in the
early 1960s, circulating stem cells that could turn into body
parts were not known to exist, so Becker's findings were not
well appreciated. (I would like to say "Science is stubborn," but
really it's a trait of the scientists themselves.)

What Becker observed was red blood cells retracing their
evolution. We all start out as a single cell, sperm and egg, which
then keeps dividing and *differentiates* into bone, heart, muscle,
nerves, and so forth. All the cells have the same genes carried
by the same chromosomes. Differentiation occurs when some
of the genes are suppressed. How the body knows to do this,
and perfectly, is officially a mystery. Becker was watching the
process in reverse: mature blood cells reverting to their original

embryonic form where they can become anything. In the case of a salamander with a severed limb, they become the various parts of the limb: regeneration. Becker called the process *dedifferentiation*—i.e., differentiation's opposite.

Another example was discovered accidentally. Becker needed blood from salamanders. He was now able to accomplish dedifferentiation in a Petri dish, by applying the same electrical currents of injury. But you don't draw blood from a salamander's arm, so he anesthetized the little amphibians, and then snipped off and discarded the top half of the heart, in order to harvest blood. The accidental part was that the heart grew back!

"Regeneration of the Ventricular Myocardium [heart muscle] in Amphibians" was the title of the article in the prestigious British journal *Nature* in 1974. The blood clot that developed to plug the salamander's bleeding heart did more: The red blood cells dedifferentiated into stem cells. That's how the heart gradually re-formed. It didn't simply knit together; rather, it grew back the missing half. While the editor of *Nature* was willing to publish this very unusual and unexpected finding (not all editors are so open-minded), Becker was not allowed to use the term "stem cells" because the concept, at the time, was just too wild and crazy. He was only allowed to say "some active cellular process" restored the lost heart muscle and that "the origin of the reparative cells and the mechanism used . . . is, as yet, unclear."

The stem cells you hear a lot about these days are those from embryos; these have the greatest potential for medical use. The first human embryonic stem cells were isolated by a team at the University of Wisconsin in 1998. Stem cells from adult mammals (particularly mice) that could transform into different types of blood cells had been known for several decades. Adults' cells that could become specific body parts — known as somatic stem cells — came along later. In adult humans, some of these pre-exist, as if in waiting, in body tissues, although it's not known where they come from.

In a more recent publication, "Induced Dedifferentiation: A Possible Alternative to Embryonic Stem Cell Transplants" in the journal *NeuroRehabilitation* (2002), Becker used a nylon fabric containing silver to enhance wound healing. Previously he had used this in people with poorly healing wounds, but used a small electrical current. This time, he believes that he has obtained dedifferentiation of mature human cells (into stem cells) without adding any electricity. Humans, while they're no match for salamanders, do have some natural regenerative powers. A child of ten years or less will regenerate an entire fingertip if the wound is not tightly covered.

Another human tissue that regenerates well is bone. That's why fractures heal. Occasionally they don't, and that's a big problem, resulting in a useless limb. It had been known since the early nineteenth century that sometimes an externally applied electric current could facilitate bone healing. Becker and others experimented with this, obtaining success with implanted electrodes. But these are inconvenient; so, building on Becker's work, an orthopedist who had worked with Becker, and an electrochemist (they had met by chance), together made a device that was external. It emitted a magnetic signal that translated into electricity at the fracture site, could be incorporated into the cast, and allowed some bones to heal that had thus far stubbornly refused to knit together. It was the first device approved by the Food and Drug Administration (in 1979) to use magnetic fields for healing.

A Blueprint for the Body

One curious thing about a salamander is that if you cut off a right foreleg, it grows back a right foreleg, proportioned appropriately, with five fingers. Remove a left hindleg, and a perfect replacement ultimately appears. How does the salamander's body keep track of exactly which parts are missing? For that matter, how does an embryo, human or animal, align itself perfectly with a head on one end and legs on the other, and each organ in just the right place? Both situations start with stem cells, which seem to know not only what to become, but where their placement within the body will be.

Back in the 1920s and 1930s, a number of scientists, including an American embryologist named Paul Weiss, proposed a morphogenetic field to explain the body's sense of orientation in space. As in the fields created by electricity and magnetism (electromagnetic fields, or EMFs), every point within the field was uniquely defined. Thus, the field pattern became a blueprint of the entire organism: a literal template for growth and development. Just as loose iron filings tossed at a magnet will align themselves along the magnet's lines of force, cells within the morphogenetic field would line up and behave appropriately for the forces at their particular points within the field.

Becker took it further, proposing that this template for life actually *was* an electromagnetic field; and, with very sensitive instruments, he measured it. On the surface of salamanders and humans, differences in electrical charge could be measured, which were consistent and changed predictably. Both species had a small back-to-front current across the head, which diminished and then reversed during anesthesia. Becker found that he could anesthetize salamanders without drugs, using only specific electrical currents (or electromagnetic fields, which would induce currents). When the field was removed, the salamander woke up. This trick was not tried on humans.

Electricity, Magnetism, and Beyond

In the chapter on hypnosis, I stated that there is no physiologic way to measure whether a subject is truly hypnotized. This is the conventional wisdom, and this is what contemporary textbooks will say. Becker found otherwise. Working with a psychologist and a physicist, "Direct Current Potentials in Hypnoanalgesia" examined the back-to-front current of human subjects as they were hypnotized. Published in the *Archives of General Psychology* in 1962, this was a study of six easily hypnotizable young men who had their cross-head currents measured with electrodes against the skin (one forehead, one back of neck) while they were brought in and out of light trance. The currents clearly diminished with attainment of the hypnotic state, similarly to anesthesia, although less pronounced. The voltage changes (voltage drives current) under hypnosis were from 0.001 to 0.005 (1 to 5 thousandths) of a volt, small but measurable.

Becker had already noted that healing is influenced by these bio-currents, and his aforementioned work on acupuncture points showed that there was an electrical reality to the points, suggesting that pain perception may be mediated by current flow. He believes that emotion, on a physiologic level, modulates the current that controls pain and healing, and thus might account for the placebo effect or even the "miracle" cures of shamans, faith healers, and saints. Unlike the vague "energy" attributed to distant healers, homeopathic remedies, or therapeutic touch, Becker's biofield is measurable and quantifiable.

The earth itself is one giant magnet, the result of molten iron spinning at its core. This allows a compass needle—which is just a tiny, free-to-rotate magnet—to assume its position: pointing north. Until 1820, magnetism and electricity were thought to be two distinct entities. Then the Danish physicist Oersted noticed that a compass needle deflected when electric current in a wire passed nearby. Now the two are wedded; each can create the other, given the right circumstances.

Life developed within the earth's magnetic field. The small electric currents Becker (and others) have recorded are entwined with the earth's field. Bacteria have magnetic sensors. Clams open their shells, in unison, in response to the earth's magnetism. Birds navigate thousands of miles using the lines of the earth's magnetic force. (Birds' primary system uses light from the sun, which they polarize—i.e., directionalize. Magnetism kicks in on cloudy days.)

In Becker's 1985 book *The Body Electric* (written with Gary Selden), the orthopedist observes: "Following the curious dogma that what we don't understand can't exist, mainstream science has dismissed psychic phenomena as delusions or hoaxes simply because they're rarer than sleep, dreams, memory, growth, pain, or consciousness, which are all inexplicable in traditional terms but are too common to be denied." Then Becker goes on to wonder if electromagnetic fields, both the ones our bodies generate and the earth's, could be a possible basis for telepathy (ESP). He believes gifted healers generate "supportive electromagnetic effects." In a second book five years later, *Cross Currents*, he bolsters this idea with research from China (not MEDLINE-accessible) where Qi Gong (again, a form of Chinese "energy" healing) is tested for its effects on an organic chemical compound that was known to change under the influence of weak EMFs. Charting the compound's behavior with an MRI scanner, a Qi Gong healer could rearrange the compound, as could a machine emitting an EMF signal. And neither needed the other's help.

Becker writes of a Russian experiment (also MEDLINE-inaccessible) on forty professional dowsers. The test premise had to do with whether finding water way below the surface may use an unconscious sense of the EMFs that water creates in the earth. The forty were outfitted with wires and magnets that might jam subtle signals to see if these would diminish skills. They did, markedly.

In fact, Becker surmises that a specific channel of biologic EMFs exists that might allow communication by waveform, particularly if people used the same frequencies. These would be biologically programmed in, and could be expected to be closest in relatives and, especially, identical twins. These are situations where telepathy, when it occurs, seems to work best.

The earth, as mentioned, has its own magnetic field (such a field surrounds any magnet), known as the geomagnetic field, and it varies a bit on the planet's surface, and is also affected by the moon's position and the sun's activity. Sometimes the field is relatively quiescent; other times it is roiled up by extra turmoil on the sun's surface. This can reach the earth as what we call a magnetic storm. If severe, these can interfere with radio and TV reception. Most go unnoticed unless, like the government's U.S. Geologic Survey, you're in the business of measuring them. Storms can last a few days, and may occur as often as two or three times a month; or there may not be any for a few months.

One problem with studying psychic powers lies in the difficulty of reproducing results. Scientific credibility depends upon the ability of independent researchers, using the same techniques, to reach the same conclusions. Becker assumes that the transmission of ESP information is akin to the way radio and TV work, and has measured, with sensitive instruments, enough electricity and magnetism emanating from living things to make this assumption interesting. Radio-type waves do not appear to be involved in telepathy. Radio reception diminishes with distance, which does not seem to be the case with ESP. What's more, subjects placed in rooms that shield these waves can still display psychic skills.

Can the earth's magnetic field, in concert with the body's innate fields, function as an information conduit? The basic electroencephalographic rhythm of the brain—the alpha waves, at eight to fourteen per second—match the rhythm of the magnetic micropulsations in the earth's field. Becker feels that this is not a coincidence. Writing in the non–MEDLINE-indexed *Journal of the American Society for Psychical Research* in 1992, Becker reported on four independent studies, presented at the 1986 meeting of the American Psychological Association, that examined ESP powers with regard to the geomagnetic field. On days when the field was relatively quiet, telepathy functioned well. But on days when the field was stirred up by the sun's activity, as in magnetic storms, the abilities fared poorly. It appeared that geomagnetic agitation interfered with the mechanism of brain-to-brain transmission.

As is ensconced in folklore, people just seem crazier when the moon is full. It's an ancient belief that celestial bodies influence behavior. Becker took the concept further and made it more specific: He studied the effects of magnetic storms (which come from the sun) on psychiatric admissions. Working with psychologist Howard Friedman, admissions to seven central New York State psychiatric hospitals were tabulated against reports on geomagnetic activity taken from the government's Fredericksburg (Virginia) Magnetic Observatory. More storm activity correlated with more psychiatric admissions, and the data were statistically significant. Their paper, "Geomagnetic Parameters and Psychiatric Hospital Admissions," was published by *Nature* in 1963.

Unheralded and Unsung

Despite publications in major journals, Becker's work has been largely unnoticed. He has often worked on his own time and without funding. Scientists are hyperfocused on molecule–molecule interactions and don't believe that electricity or magnetism are significant. Unexplainable results don't seem to prompt new ways of looking at things. A medical student assigned to spend time in my office told me of research in which she had participated. Chick and quail embryos had their nascent, developing regions of tissue, known as somites, rearranged or removed. Somehow, the little embryos knew what was supposed to be where, and things redeveloped in their proper places. The researchers could not figure out how, but remarked that the teeny birds could alter their somite count "to one more compatible with the host's pattern" and that "the location and size of somites could also be adjusted by the host." To Becker, this is a clear example of the embryo's electromagnetic template in action.

How proteins fold—i.e., configure themselves—is another area of mystery. Conformation to an electronic blueprint, an unexplored avenue, could explain it. Becker even believes that DNA's helical form results from its evolution within a similarly shaped field.

In a 1999 study (in *The Journal of Neuroscience*), embryonic human brain stem cells were transplanted into the brains of adult rats. The human cells then proceeded to migrate, as if they were rats' stem cells, to the precise sites where they would be needed, where they became the appropriate cell types. The authors call this migration a response to "guidance cues and signals," but aren't more specific.

The implications of a morphogenetic field invite speculation. Is it formed at the union of sperm and egg, or does it somehow pre-exist? Rupert Sheldrake, a British Ph.D. biochemist who has written a number of delightful books on the unexplained powers of the mind, believes that the field is not a classical electromagnetic one, but rather a variant not yet known to physics. He postulates that similar fields, as from the same species, resonate with one another, a possible explanation for shared traits, even a collective unconscious. Sheldrake sees out-of-body experiences as those of a morphogenetic field leaving a body and returning. Phantom limbs—the perception of a missing arm or leg as still being there, even feeling pain—can be viewed as a whole-body field effect.

Becker does not know where the fields come from. He has measured them, even mapped them out in amphibians and humans, at least in their direct-current format. His salamander's field map, taken with surface electrodes, was published in *Institute of Radio Engineers Transactions in Medical Electronics* in 1960. He believes there is a dual nervous system: the conventional one, where impulses travel along nerves, and a more primitive version, where direct currents travel alongside nerves and transmit different kinds of information.

As a matter of fact, most of the cells within the nervous system don't conduct impulses. Known as glial cells, we are taught that they are there to "support" the nerve cells. This could be structural support, protection from infection, or to make something a nerve needs; but, largely, we don't really know what they do. Which is odd, because glial cells are much more numerous than nerve cells: almost half the brain's volume is taken up by glial cells. (They are smaller than nerve cells, so despite greater numbers they don't occupy more space.) Becker thinks one of their functions is to conduct direct-current electricity—a primitive nervous system that augments and completes our more developed, conventional version.

A recent publication in *Nature* from the University of Rochester suggests that epilepsy may be triggered by glial cells, rather than by nerve cells, as is commonly believed.

Meanwhile, no one is currently pursuing Dr. Becker's line of research.

Nineteen

The God Helmet and the Temporal Lobes: The Work of Michael A. Persinger

Michael A. Persinger, Ph.D., is a professor of neuroscience at Laurentian University in Sudbury, Ontario, Canada, a good two hundred miles from Toronto up in the mining country north of Lake Huron. He has been there since 1971. A MED-LINE search using "persinger ma" (October 2005) brings up almost three hundred publications he has authored or co-authored. Nevertheless, the medical colleagues with whom I rub shoulders on a day-to-day basis at an American medical school are unfamiliar with him and his work.

He was already a chemist and a physicist when he decided to become a psychologist. But he combined his science training with his study of human behavior, figuring that brain biology had to be correlated with emotions, fears (real or imagined), and most other aspects of psychopathology that afflict us. While most of the research in this field looks at the diagrammable dance of the brain's molecules, Persinger realized (as did Robert Becker) that the brain was an electric and magnetic organ as well, capable of transmitting and responding to electrical and magnetic fields. This energy is depicted in waveforms that traverse and affect the brain, as do the individual molecules that fall under their influence.

The Rhythms of Brain and Earth

An electroencephalogram (EEG) records minute rhythmic voltages from the scalp. These are the orchestrations of nerve firings, conducted from deeper within the brain. Why, exactly, do nerves fire in synchronous rhythms? We don't really know. In the heart, all the muscle fibers contract in unison so that the heart can function as a pump. Why the resting brain "beats" is a mystery.

Can one look at the brain as an electrical organ? Karl Pribram felt that the nerves' connections (synapses) trafficked electricity in addition to molecular messengers. Becker, as mentioned, believes that the abundant glial cells constitute a primitive nervous system that uses direct electrical currents. Persinger feels that all levels of the brain are responsive to the sea of electricity and magnetism generated by the body and by the earth, and this opens many possibilities.

Persinger's work has been particularly attentive to the effects of the earth's geomagnetic field on behavior. As mentioned, the earth is a big magnet. Living things, by virtue of the electric currents they generate, are little magnets. Little magnets are affected by big magnets and, to a much lesser extent, by each other. Persinger has published research linking variations in the earth's natural magnetic properties to such diverse happenings as commercial air crashes, UFO sightings, visions of religious figures, sudden infant deaths, poltergeists and haunted homes, apparitions of the dead, and impending earthquakes.

Before elaborating on these, a few words about the earth's fields. There is a constancy, which makes compasses reliable; and then there are fluctuations, small but measurable. These include a pulsatile component, at about the same frequency as the brain's basic alpha waves (Becker considered this "breathing with the earth"), and many minor ripples, at intensities similar to the body's own fields. The weather, particularly thunder and lightning storms; the moon, whether it's day or night; and energy radiating from the sun—all affect the earth's field. So although it's always there, it is going to vary at different times and places.

And that becomes one basis for Persinger's studies. Most of this work was published in the MEDLINE-indexed journal *Perceptual and Motor Skills,* usually with one or two colleagues. As I cite it, I'll just give the year.

- From records of commercial airline crashes (2004), 373 mishaps from 1940 through 2002 were examined. These were attributed to one of four problems: computer error, pilot error, mechanical failures, and, of course, unknown factors. Persinger looked at global geomagnetic activity on the days of the crashes and for three days before and after. He found significantly greater activity on the days of pilot or computer failures, but not when the problem was mechanical or unknown. He hypothesizes that "some factor or factors associated with relative increases in geomagnetic activity may affect complex electronic systems composed of either silica (computer) or carbon (brain) aggregates."

- In "Relations Between UFO Reports within the Uinta Basin and Local Seismicity" (1985), Persinger and seismologist John Derr looked at seismic (earthquake-type) activity in a mountainous area of northeast Utah and related it to UFO sightings. There was a correlation within about a hundred miles of the activity, but not beyond that. The epicenters here were mere ground vibrations rather than knock-the-cups-off-your-shelf earthquakes, and as they shifted through the area, so did the UFO reports. Persinger believes the strains between the earth's tectonic plates (which can culminate in a quake) generate electrical and magnetic fields that cause both distortions in human perceptions and in the earth's atmosphere.

- In 1989 and in 2001, Persinger and John Derr examined sightings of the Virgin Mary, and related them to electromagnetic changes in the terrain. First, at a Coptic Christian church in Zeitoun, near Cairo, Egypt, hundreds of thousands of people reported seeing apparitions of the Virgin Mary from 1968 to 1971. Photos of these showed "irregular blobs of light," according to Persinger. These were of two types: small, rapidly moving lights, perceived by onlookers as doves, or a persisting, rounded glow at the top of the church, visualized as the Virgin Mary. (Pictures of these are available on Web sites, which is to say, not from the medical literature, and these posted photos, for whatever it's worth, show a pretty good rendition of doves and the Virgin Mary.)

  An unusual tenfold increase in seismic activity was noted some two hundred miles away. While this is a considerable distance, the concept of linking naturally generated electromagnetic forces with "luminous phenomena" is interesting.

- Subsequently, mid-1990s reports of religious experiences at a Canadian town halfway between Toronto and Ottawa prompted a study. The enlightened area was near a hilltop adjacent to an open-pit magnetite mine (magnetite is an iron ore from which the first magnets were made). Water poured continuously into the mine, which increases the strain on earthquake-prone land masses. Seismic epicenters drifted closer to the hilltop. These unusual "geophysical" conditions made the spot ripe, theoretically, for unusual human perception. Persinger and co-author Lynn Suess were able to associate increases in geomagnetic activity, as well as measurable changes in ambient magnetic fields, with the experiencers' reports.

In both of these "luminous phenomena" events, the belief is that pressure along fault lines generates electromagnetic activity to which some people's brains are sensitive. Whether the perceptions are projections from within the brain, or an enhanced ability to see what normally isn't seeable—that's another question. Persinger recently told writer Mary Roach[13] that he can't rule out the latter possibility.

• The brain's pineal gland secretes a hormone called melatonin, which regulates some other hormones and also enhances the immune system. The pineal, in the midline not far behind the eyes, is light-sensitive. More melatonin is made at night (which is why it's sometimes used as a sleeping pill), and its production is affected by other types of electromagnetic waves as well. Persinger and colleague R. P. O'Connor hypothesized that specific ranges of geomagnetic activity that cause sudden decreases in nocturnal melatonin might also precipitate sudden infant death, usually a nighttime phenomenon. Their 1997 publication found certain ranges of geomagnetism to correlate with cases of sudden infant death.

In a follow-up paper in 2001, the two looked at occurrences of sudden infant deaths and of hospital admissions of adults with electrical cardiac rhythm disturbances, postulating that geomagnetic

13 Roach, M. *Spook*, p 221. New York: W.W. Norton, 2005.

blips might be a common denominator. They found that both conditions do vary in tandem with the earth's geomagnetism.

- Poltergeists are literally "noisy ghosts." Persinger (1986) observed their association with strange noises and movements of objects, as well as "electromagnetic peculiarities" and odd human behaviors. Some geographic locales had a lot of cases; others had none. Persinger and Livingston Gearhart, a professor of music at the State University of New York at Buffalo, found that these hauntings seemed to parallel sudden increases in global geomagnetic activity. Working with geomagnetic records and with reports of poltergeists, similar patterns were observed in Europe and North America: Poltergeist episodes were more likely on or just before days of geomagnetic turbulence.

Try This On

But the singular thing for which Persinger is best known, media-wise, is his electromagnetic helmet. This is a motorcycle-style hard hat fitted with coils and wires that deliver a variety of signals through the brain. These are imperceptible, low-frequency, low-intensity waveforms that can simulate the earth's own fields, and can be adjusted to create different types of brain "experiences." Volunteers so outfitted sit in a sensory-deprivation chamber (it's soundproof, and volunteers' eyes are covered) and may feel relaxed, see God, encounter ghosts or space aliens, go "out-of-body," believe they have lived before, sense a vague "presence," or have no such visions.

Reporters have called this contraption "The UFO Machine" (*Spectrum* magazine) or "The God Helmet" (*Saturday Night* magazine), or referred to the experience as "This is Your Brain on God" (*Wired* magazine) or "God on the Brain" (BBC Two). Here is a sampling of helmet studies — or "transcerebral, weak, complex magnetic fields," as Persinger refers to them:

- (1996) Twenty-one otherwise normal young men and women who believed they had lived a past life were compared to fifty-two who did not. Persinger's surveys of students at his Canadian university consistently show that 25 percent of students believe that they have lived before. Surveys of Americans show the same percentage. Under stimulation for thirty minutes, the "believers" were more likely to experience spinning, tingling, detachment from their bodies, and intrusions of thoughts not their own. Women were more likely than men to be so stimulated. Right-brain tweaking brought more results than left-brain. Persinger uses fields that could occur in the environment under some conditions, and finds some brains more susceptible.

- (1997) Three-minute magnetic bursts were applied to fifteen volunteers and to one "exceptional" subject, chosen because he felt that he could sense people's health problems by looking at their photographs. Nine of the fifteen sensed a "presence," a sort of "you are not alone" feeling. The special subject sensed presences rather easily, including the times when the fields were turned on without his knowing. Persinger believes that the "sensed presence" is a common phenomenon, which includes religious experiences of God or angels, as well as spirit visitations.

- (2000) A forty-five-year-old man who had previously been troubled by a haunt experience had the haunting reproduced in Persinger's laboratory within ten minutes of a field application to the right-brain hemisphere; he even saw the apparition, and said that this "synthetic" ghost was much like the one that had found him on its own.

The three previous studies were reported in *Perceptual and Motor Skills*. The next two are from the *International Journal of Neuroscience*.

- (2001) People were told an emotionally charged story and then given a recap, either accurate or inaccurate. Different types of complex magnetic fields were fed in as well. One week later, subjects were asked to retell the story. The combination of right-hemisphere stimulation plus the inaccurate summary produced three times as many false memories as did either of these alone.

- (2005) In this one, Persinger and associates waited for squalls of natural geomagnetic activity and then zapped in the weak fields. This turned out to be a more effective way of eliciting a sense of a supernatural presence or sentient being. The question, then, is to what extent turbulence in the electromagnetic weather brings out this perception in people who, by virtue of a little electrical instability in the right side of their brains, are susceptible.

Persinger claims that eighty percent of the people he's helmet-tested have some sort of altered consciousness during the trial, usually a sensed presence. Generally, the experiences are pleasant; occasionally, they're frightening or unpleasant, or they may include a sensation of someone grabbing you. The *Wired* reporter tried on the hat and then conjured up a few childhood memories, including one of his girlfriend when he was fourteen. *Saturday Night*'s writer had some pleasant, kaleidoscope-type visual hallucinations. The BBC's correspondent told of the helmet experience of one of Britain's most renowned atheists: His breathing and his arms and legs felt different; he did not find God.

Persinger's helmet work is hard to confirm, to the extent that it requires his equipment. A Swedish team visited his laboratory, had the equipment demonstrated to them, and then were sent a portable version to try. They concluded that "Sensed presence and mystical experiences are predicted by suggestibility, not by the application of transcranial weak magnetic fields." They found that "individuals with a high degree of openness to unusual experiences" who, like good hypnosis candidates, were suggestible, were more likely to report an experience. Persinger felt that the researchers used his machinery incorrectly; it does appear that their attempt was made in good faith.

The Temporal Lobe Has Tales to Tell

The electromagnetic stimuli under Persinger's command are usually directed toward the brain's temporal lobes. To the extent that the brain, from the side, resembles a boxing glove, the temporal lobe would be the thumb. This is an interesting part of the brain. The more mundane parts control things like movement, sensation, vision, breathing. But stimulation of the temporal lobe, as neurosurgeon Wilder Penfield did in his epilepsy patients, evokes memories, emotions, hallucinations of sights, sounds, or smells, or déjà vu. British neurologist Adam Zeman, writing in the *New England Journal of Medicine* (January 13, 2005), in a piece called "Tales From the Temporal Lobes," calls them "a monumental library equipped to catalogue, store, and retrieve the experiences of a lifetime." He points out how disturbances in their function, such as epilepsy, can create amnesia, incongruous emotions, or even out-of-body experiences.

Thus, some "paranormal" phenomena can be attributed to seizure activity within the temporal lobes. Temporal lobe attacks are currently called partial seizures; consciousness may or may not be lost. They've been also called psychomotor or temporal lobe epilepsy. These attacks are different from generalized seizures, which result in whole-body-shaking, fall-to-the-floor unconsciousness. A partial, or temporal lobe-based, seizure might trigger such a full-blown convulsion, or it might merely cause episodes of bizarre behavior with amnesia rather than a classic epileptic fit. Psychiatric texts make mention of this.

Most patients with partial epilepsy, however, don't go into altered states. In a textbook-quoted[14] study, twenty-five percent of 414 such patients exhibited changes in psychic function during an attack. Often these are combined with abnormal movements; co-existing generalized seizures may also be part of the picture. The electroencephalogram is usually awry. The diagnosis of a true seizure disorder is more or less evident.

When psychic symptoms do occur, they may include déjà vu, illusions, memory recall, sexual or emotional items, personality changes, body image distortions, or a sense of a presence nearby. These were listed in a recent paper by neurologist R. Mark Sadler and Susan Rahey in the journal *Epilepsia* (2004). They had come upon three patients with medically diagnosed temporal lobe epilepsy who had precognition—a sense of knowing what's about to happen—at the beginning of their seizure. Déjà vu was combined with it. (It may be that if you think you've seen it before, you'd also think you would know what was

14 *Principles of Neurology* (6th ed., 1997) p. 322.

going to happen next, but Sadler believes there's some difference.) The conclusion is that precognition (prescience) "can be
a symptom of temporal lobe-originating seizures."

Back in 1981, a Harvard study of twelve patients referred
for dissociative-type psychiatric problems found all twelve to
have some abnormality in EEG's taken from their temporal
lobes. Dissociation comes up frequently in this book; it is
among medicine's most bizarre syndromes. Seven of the Harvard patients had multiple personality disorder, and five had
possession issues. Only three of the twelve had bona fide con-
vulsive symptoms sufficient to label as epilepsy, but the author
feels that all twelve probably qualify for this diagnosis, and
that the psychiatric symptoms may result from temporal lobe
seizure activity.

Persinger and others have made a connection between paranormal beliefs and partial (temporal lobe) epilepsy. A 1985
paper by Persinger looked at university students and correlated temporal lobe signs—things that could be construed as
seizure activity, like déjà vu—with students' reports of paranormal experiences. This was a "normal population," not people diagnosed with seizures. He concludes that "mystical or
paranormal experiences are associated with transient electrical
foci within the temporal lobe of the human brain."

A Canadian team at the University of Windsor, Ontario, publishing in the *British Journal of Clinical Psychology* in 1996, also
sampling university students, found the same relationship. A
more recent work from the department of psychology at the University of Arizona is entitled "Near-Death Experiences and the
Temporal Lobe." They found more epilepsy-like electroencephalographic action in the left temporal lobes of people who
had described near-death experiences and concluded that

"individuals who have had such experiences are physiologically distinct from the general population."

Standard medical texts have interesting things to say about the temporal lobes. In *Principles of Neurology* (6th ed., 1997), these regions coordinate sensations, emotions, and behavior, are continuously active, and can be seen as a seat of self-awareness and even of consciousness itself. In *Synopsis of Psychiatry* (9th ed., 2003), schizophrenia is mentioned as a possible consequence of temporal lobe seizure activity; in some studies, seven percent of temporal lobe epilepsy patients have associated schizophrenia.

So Persinger's basic thesis is that people's temporal lobes vary in sensitivity to electricity and magnetism in the environment. Some of us, due to an innate instability in this part of the brain, may be affected by naturally occurring "geophysical" events. Persinger's helmet is made to recreate these; its emanations are designed to mimic signals that could originate in nature.

The Hills and the Homes are Alive

Persinger has also examined the effects of fields emitted from man-made devices. In two separate reports in *Perceptual and Motor Skills* in 2001, paranormal experiences were linked to such exposures. In the first, a female teenager complained of "nightly visitations by a sentient being." These involved vibrations of the bed and a sense of a presence that her body could feel, including sexually. This is reminiscent of Mrs. A. (chapter 7: Intimate Demons); both women felt that they had had intercourse with "a force," although the teenager attributed this to the Holy Spirit, rather than the devil. Persinger found that an electric clock sat eight inches away from the girl's head as she slept. When the clock was removed, the visitations stopped. The girl rapidly became the province of psychiatrists, and no further follow-up was available.

The second report concerned a small house where a couple suffered waves of fear, apparitions, and a sensed presence. These included seeing shadows on the wall, sounds of whispering, and feeling something touching their feet. Persinger measured the house to be "electronically dense," packed with electrical appliances and electronic equipment, and compounded by earth currents and poor grounding. He believes that these, plus an inherent susceptibility of the people involved, created the haunting. In both of these reports, the "sensed presence" is interpreted culturally (religious; ghost).

Persinger believes that the land in some areas is just naturally more alive, electronically speaking. This is particularly true over earthquake faults. People living in these areas, then, may be more likely to experience the bizarre. Some may be genetically prone, due to instability within the temporal lobes.

Persinger also believes that it is not an accident that lightning and thunderstorms, which whip up an area's electromagnetism, are associated in folklore and in literature with the paranormal.

Telepathy, Too

Persinger has another line of interest: information acquisition. While he explains away some paranormal phenomena via interactions of waveforms and temporal lobe hotspots, he has also worked with subjects who had strong telepathic skills. In chapter 3 (the Remote Viewing section), I mentioned his work with a New York artist named Ingo Swann, who could reliably discern photographs within sealed envelopes in another room. He has also studied another man, also middle-aged, named Sean Harribance, who can do the same. Both are discussed in "The Neuropsychiatry of Paranormal Experiences" in *The Journal of Neuropsychiatry* in 2001.

Their abilities were studied as they "received" information from within a room shielded from sound and most electromagnetic activity, known as a Faraday cage. Cell phones and radios won't work, as these are higher frequency waves (half a million cycles per second and up). Very low-frequency waves, ten cycles per second or less, pass through. These are the type generated in nature or by living things. The earth's magnetic field also gets through, although it might be somewhat distorted, so that, for instance, a compass will work.

How was information transmitted to these two subjects? Very low-frequency waves? Embedded into and conducted through the geomagnetic field? In the experiment cited earlier, complex waveforms generated by a Windows operating system "jammed" Mr. Swann's reception, suggesting that some type of wave transmission is involved.

Persinger believes, as do others who research these sorts of things, that telepathy works best when the ambient electromagnetics are relatively quiet. Nighttime, absence of magnetic storms, and the subject's being free of distractions would be examples. On the other hand, visions, ghosts, or "presences" might be enhanced by stronger geomagnetic activity.

A Better Question

Why sensed presences or mystical experiences can be conjured up at all—by seizures, by hypnosis, by psychedelic drugs, by Persinger's machine, or by suggestion—is another question. Even if people are suggestible enough to "see" strange things if they are told to do so, there are still areas of our brains, particularly in the temporal lobes, that, when activated electrically, give us strange senses of time and place. This is clear just from studies on epilepsy.

What are these regions of our central nervous system doing there? Did they evolve? Are they adaptive? Are they remnants of a more primitive time in our history? Persinger sees them as a way of connecting mankind together. His term "sensed presence" describes a generic feeling of not being alone, which can be interpreted culturally as anything from God to space aliens to dragons. If you recall Stanley Milgram's "obedience to authority" experiment, it appeared that such obedience was more or less a basic element of human nature. Is it mediated through these same brain regions? Is this what allows humankind to work together under the direction of a leader, spiritual or political, and to pursue common goals that would not be attainable as individuals? If so, that would certainly be adaptive.

I previously mentioned that hallucinations, particularly auditory, can be normal in some contexts. A 1976 book by Princeton psychologist Julian Jaynes, *The Origin of Consciousness in the Breakdown of the Bicameral Mind*, theorizes that our earlier, more primitive, brains, prior to 1000 B.C., were more like the brains of today's schizophrenics or mystics, seeing visions, hearing voices—i.e., sensing a presence. Jaynes uses archaeological data and writings like the Iliad to bolster his idea. He theorizes that these "hallucinations," attributed to gods, were widespread and considered normal: They directed behavior and bound people socially, and then faded as written language developed, which could do the same. (Jaynes feels that modern-day possession states, hypnotic suggestibility, and schizophrenia are throwbacks to this primeval mind.) Perhaps we've retained a bit of madness that once served a purpose.

Persinger believes that the neuroscience of unexplainable phenomena will ultimately decipher them, and that words like "parapsychology" or "paranormal" will no longer need to exist. He funds his work himself, with an occasional private grant. It is hard to imagine that he has placed 298 entries into the medical literature without being on to something.

$\mathcal{T}$wenty

Perspective II: Witches in the Waiting Room, and Everywhere

In 1993, Dr. David M. Eisenberg of the Harvard Medical School published what would become a landmark study in the *New England Journal of Medicine:* "Unconventional Medicine in the United States: Prevalence, Costs, and Patterns of Use." Eisenberg used a telephone survey of over fifteen hundred adults to conclude that unconventional (later "alternative") therapies were a real part of the medical lives of over a third of our patients.

"Unconventional" included acupuncture, chiropractic, massage, prayer, hypnosis, and a variety of other things. That patients were into these things doesn't sound surprising now; but in 1993, alternative medicine was sufficiently alien to the medical profession that most of us didn't know what was going on before our eyes. Eisenberg's paper forced us to notice; a flood of letters to the *New England Journal* made it obvious that some doctors had already noticed and didn't think alternative medicine was a bad thing. Even physicians who weren't enthusiastic about the medical benefits of such alternative care realized that they were being left out of the loop: Patients were availing themselves of these therapies and not telling their doctors.

And so alternative medicine was launched. It became okay to mention it to your doctor. It became okay to look at studies of alternative therapies to see what they could and could not do. It even became okay for the National Institutes of Health to make research money available to study these therapies further. Alternative medicine was out of the closet.

As research accumulated, some alternative treatments turned mainstream. Acupuncture was vetted for at least a few conditions. Chiropractic manipulation, in some studies, provided more low-back pain relief at one week than conventional therapy (although there was no difference at one month). Certain herbal remedies contained active substances that really did work. The unconventional, bolstered by data, became conventional.

The alternative overlaps the paranormal, as both are incompletely understood. That is why some of Eisenberg's unconventional therapies comprise chapters in this book. But there is another similarity: Patients who have had paranormal experiences or hold paranormal beliefs, which may be significant enough to impact their health, are unlikely to share this with their doctors. As Eisenberg pointed out, a great deal goes on in front of our medical noses that we don't know about.

My patients have no idea that I have an interest in the paranormal. My general medical practice is rather conventional. I don't do alternative medicine. Whatever reaches me in the way of a bizarre patient experience does so by chance; I don't look for it. Since I've started writing this book, however, co-workers who know of my interest will sometimes share something relevant with me, and I will, rarely, ask a patient about the subject. Let me tell you what has come my way over the years:

- Turning the pages of my local newspaper one morning, I see that a young woman who has been a patient of mine is being sued for divorce and child custody by her husband because . . . she is a witch. Literally. According to the paper, the husband would be awakened in the middle of the night by noises, and find his wife robed and chanting and unresponsive to him. If true, this is what a psychiatrist would call dissociation, possibly a multiple personality disorder, or something called a fugue state. My patient, in the article, denied any such goings-on. I did see her in the office about two years later, with her mom, and didn't bring up the news item; neither did she. Of course, at the time I didn't know I'd be writing this book.

- Recently, another patient came to see me who I knew had been an acquaintance of this first woman. I asked her what she thought. She hadn't seen the other woman in years, but her sense was that this had happened in the context of a bitter divorce, with the husband and his mother vying for custody of the child. In messy divorces these days, anything goes; why not accusations of witchcraft? My present patient did say that my former patient had been a serious witchcraft hobbyist, but that she thought the reported accusations were greatly exaggerated.

  Then she added that she, too, was a fairly serious witchcraft hobbyist.

- I found out, in a casual conversation with a colleague, that a female resident whom I had trained considered herself a witch. And her mother was a witch too. I can say that none of these three women had anything about them that struck me as peculiar, other-worldly, or in any way out of the ordinary. In fact, these three seemed pretty well-adjusted.

- At a clinic where I teach, the same clinic where years earlier the banker who "died on time" had been a patient, a nurse told me that many of our patients there were witches, some professional. Naively, I asked what the difference was between a serious witch-craft hobbyist and a professional witch. It turns out that our clinic's professional witches get *paid* for their services. Yikes.

  The nurse explaining this to me had a master's degree in applied anthropology, from which her interest derived. As I asked some questions about witchcraft, I ascertained that our practitioners were multi-ethnic, and practicing different types of the craft. (The term "witchcraft" encompasses many sects and variations; for simplicity, I'm using the word in its general sense.) Then another clinic nurse I'll call Angela happened by, and the anthropologist nurse said "Why don't you just ask Angela? She's a witch."

  Who knew? So Angela and I went into my office, where she was happy to talk to me. Her calling began as a teenager, when she real-ized that she had telepathic abilities. It ran in her family: Her mater-nal grandmother was a witch, her mother was not. All I had known was that Angela was an ordinary (i.e., regular) nurse.

  In other words, I go to work as a physician every day, and I'm sur-rounded by witches. I just never knew it. I suspect that my colleagues' patients are no different. Not to mention some of my colleagues and co-workers.

- Other things cross my medical path. A well-dressed, seventyish woman who is always a little anxious and depressed volunteers the information that her divorced daughter has taken up with a new boyfriend, whom she met on the Internet. The medical student also in the room knows of my interests; the patient does not. Perhaps she feels that we look sympathetic and willing to listen. According to my patient, this boyfriend "has powers." He hypnotizes her two-year-old grandchild to where the little boy tells his grandma "Don't look at me!" He defrosts bacon by putting the package in water and staring at it intently. "It pops right up to the top, defrosted," she says, looking right at me as if to say "see what I have to put up with!"

• I ask a seventy-year-old woman, whose husband is in the hospital, for a phone number where I can reach her. She takes out a business card and writes the number on the back. The front of her card says "Psychic Reader."

• A schizophrenic patient I oversee with a resident in training at the university's family practice center tells the resident physician that she believes her illness is the result of witchcraft.

• Years ago, I made an unannounced house call to a Hispanic clinic patient who had signed herself out of the hospital two months earlier. She had been admitted for a lung problem, and sputum had been collected during her stay for culture in the hospital laboratory. Now, her sputum was growing a germ that looked like tuberculosis. (It can take about six weeks to grow tuberculosis in cultures.) The woman was in her fifties, with a cough, a horrible-looking chest X-ray, and twenty or thirty pounds of lost weight. When simpler tests had failed to make a diagnosis, a lung biopsy was the next step. She wouldn't take it.

Since tuberculosis is a public health problem, I decided to go to her home with bottles of pills for her to take, if she would, and materials to test the rest of her family. Even if she didn't want treatment herself, surely she would allow testing of the others in the house, which included children. After some deliberation as I stood at the door, the family let me in.

I didn't know if the woman would be dead or alive. She had looked pretty sick two months before. But now she looked great! All the weight had returned, and she claimed to feel just fine. She laughed at the idea of swallowing the pills I'd brought. Then the family had a conference and decided to let me in on what had happened. After leaving the hospital, she had gone to a "witch doctor," who gave her some leaves in a jar, which cured her. Only she didn't even ingest these leaves; she simply placed the jar under her bed.

Everyone in the house tested negative. It was likely that her germ wasn't actually tuberculosis, but something related and more benign. However, her X-ray changes two months earlier had been striking and indicated a serious lung problem, one that would not have been expected to resolve quickly by itself. And the woman, having departed from the ranks of conventional medicine, was not going to get a follow-up film. Another day in the practice of medicine, where not everything you see makes sense.

• At the university where I teach, I overhear our social worker commenting that he's been subpoenaed to testify in a child custody trial; he had been seeing the family for counseling. The child's father was a member of a local Long Island satanic cult. He wouldn't give the six year old, who was diabetic, his insulin, claiming that his cult's powers were all the child needed. (He understandably lost custody of the child.)

Then the social worker, seeing my interest, volunteered a personal story. It seems that he has an identical twin brother. Once, while this social worker was delivering a lecture, a sudden severe knee pain, for no ostensible reason, arrived with such force that he had to stop lecturing. His twin brother, at that very moment as best as they could piece it together later, had been hit by a car.

The doctors I train and work with come from all over the world. Writing this book, it was easy to ask about, say, reincarnation beliefs in their native lands. As expected, Christians and Moslems subscribed to an afterlife, but not one on this earth. Hindus accepted reincarnation, but remained preoccupied with the hassles of this life rather than some other one.

When I asked a doctor from Cameroon, in Africa, about his attitudes toward reincarnation, he smiled and said "I am my great-grandfather." While Cameroon is predominantly Christian (as is this doctor), tribal ways are somewhat retained, and newborns are taken to the local medicine person, who proclaims who they are (i.e., who they used to be). Usually it's a former member of their own family, but I was told that, about 30 percent of the time, it's a "newcomer."

One of my colleagues is a Coptic Christian from Egypt. Having written about the sightings above a church in Zeitoun, Egypt, I asked her if she had ever heard anything about this. Well, she had actually been there! She had been a child of about nine and had gone with her mother. She had seen the doves, but was afraid of seeing the Virgin Mary and looked away. Her mother, and everyone else who was there, did see the Virgin, and the people surrounding the church saw her, I was told, from different angles, appropriate for where they were standing (like a hologram).

Her mother had an umbilical hernia at the time — a two-inch in diameter opening where her navel should have been that allowed for a bulging sphere of innards pushing through. They stayed at the church until four A.M. and then went home. When her mother awoke the next day, her hernia was gone. The open hole had been replaced by intact scar tissue. (This is not something that would happen under the rules of medical normalcy.) My colleague is extremely level-headed and competent. She practiced obstetrics in Egypt before coming here. As far as she is concerned, a miracle had been wrought upon her mother, and nothing will ever convince her otherwise.

This is reminiscent of an account by American surgeon Alexis Carrel, who won the Nobel Prize in medicine in 1912 for a method of surgically attaching blood vessels. In 1903, he wrote *The Voyage to Lourdes,* in which he recounted a healing miracle he witnessed when a dying, tuberculous teenager returned to life before his very eyes. Carrel went as a skeptic, and returned as a believer.

An emergency-room physician at my university gives a lecture on domestic violence. He makes the point that it's quite common, but you have to ask the patient about it; they don't usually volunteer this information. When he's lectured around the country, emergency-room doctors often claim never to have seen a case. They never asked. At the clinic, we did the following study: Patients were randomly seen in a room that had several posters about domestic violence on display and by a physician wearing a pin that suggested interest in the subject. Other patients were seen in a different room under usual conditions. During the study period, four of 148 women in the first room spontaneously came forth with stories of abuse. None of the 173 patients in the second room mentioned anything. (These numbers are statistically significant.)

The point is, our patients suffer domestic violence, use alternative medicine, and have paranormal experiences. If we don't know about it, it's because we're not interested. But we should be interested, because these things can affect health.

An old friend of mine, whom I ran into after many years of separation, told me the following story after he heard I was writing this book. His father died in 1975. Two days after the death, my friend got into his car, which, strangely, would not start. Suddenly he saw his father sitting in the passenger seat, real as life yet transparent like a ghost. The father spoke, reassuring his son that he was still with him. The father also advised giving something in his apartment—a potted fern—to the next-door neighbor. My friend had never been to this apartment (his dad had just moved in recently), and didn't know of the plant or the neighbor. Soon the father disappeared, and my friend was able to start the car. The plant and the neighbor were a reality. When my friend appeared at her door with the fern and told the neighbor that his father wanted her to have it, she said "Your father was a remarkable man."

Stories like this have no scientific value. They're just anecdotes, common as witches on Halloween (or in my office). You could collect thousands of similar experiences. It's impossible, at this date, to verify whether my friend acquired information he truly did not have. I bring it up for a different reason: *Ten years* elapsed before my friend told another living soul.

It is unfortunate that most people need to conceal something so common and so normal as a paranormal experience. If we don't understand such things now, sooner or later we will. Hiding them is a burden and a scientific step backward. I'd like to see science and medicine take them more seriously and study them as any naturally occurring phenomena would be studied.

In a 1980 study published in the *American Journal of Psychiatry,* University of Florida psychiatrist Stanley Dean and colleagues surveyed psychiatry professors and residents-in-training, other medical faculty, and medical-school deans. The question was "Should psychic studies be included in psychiatric education?" More than half said yes. In the paper's discussion, the authors state that "Our results indicate a high incidence of conviction among deans of medical schools and psychiatric educators that many psychic phenomena may be a reality, psychic powers are present in most or all of us, nonmedical factors play an important part in the healing process, and, above all, studies of psychic phenomena should be included in psychiatric education. . . ."

Psychic phenomena are not easily studied. Marilyn Schlitz, Ph.D., research director of the California-based Institute for Noetic Sciences, is one of the few alternative medicine researchers who get NIH grants. She and her colleagues have done a lot of work with what they call distant intentionality: Can the intentions of one person create any physiologic changes in a second person some distance away? This is the basic premise of distant healing.

The setup consists of taking couples, often related, like husband and wife, and placing one member in a soundproof, electromagnetically shielded room, while the other member sits outside of this box in a nearby room. The outer person, let's say the husband, sees a closed-circuit TV screen, on which live images of the inside person, the wife here, are occasionally projected. He thinks about his wife when he sees these images. Meanwhile the wife is having her skin conductance measured. This is essentially a measure of perspiration, evoked by barely perceptible emotional responses. Lie-detector testing uses the same principle.

Thus, if the husband thinks of his wife, and the wife reacts with a minute amount of emotion, this is measurable, objectively. (It's sort of like the superstition of your ears turning red or ringing when people are talking about you.) When Marilyn Schlitz places the couple in their appropriate stations and records the data, distant intentionality—the mental influence of one person on another—is consistently real and measurable. Schlitz designs and conducts the experiments out of a thesis that distant intentionality exists.

But when a colleague of hers, who is skeptical about this claim, does precisely the same experiment, no correlation can be demonstrated. They work with couples who are randomly assigned to either researcher; the same equipment is used. When the believer is the observer, distant intentionality happens, consistently. When the nonbeliever observes, no connection is found, consistently. So the results are consistent by researcher, albeit inconsistent when both examiners' findings are lumped together.

Can the attitude of the onlooker affect the outcome? Is this a peculiarity of psychic research? What happens, for instance, if you study angina pectoris, the squeezing, choking pain one gets when heart muscle isn't getting enough blood, threatening a heart attack?

Harvard physician Herbert Benson published a paper in the *New England Journal of Medicine* in 1979: "Angina Pectoris and the Placebo Effect." As I've mentioned previously, close to 40 percent of people who think they've been treated improve, even if the treatment consisted of little sugar pills. Benson reviewed five therapies for angina, all of which looked promising at first, but all of which were subsequently discarded for inefficacy.

These included Vitamin E, two medications, and two surgical procedures. All were found to be about 80 percent effective in initial reports. Often the parameters of effect were not just subjective, but included measurable entities like exercise tolerance, reduced nitroglycerine usage, or favorable electrocardiogram changes. What these positive studies had in common was their authors' enthusiastic belief that the treatments would be useful.

When follow-up studies were done by physicians who were not so sure that these things worked, the same treatments had no effect beyond that of sham treatment. All five therapies were abandoned. They had worked when the observer believed they would work; they failed when the observer assumed they would fail. Benson cites a reference quoting a prominent nineteenth-century French physician: "You should treat as many patients as possible with the new drugs while they still have the power to heal."

So belief in something affects outcome, whether you study people feeling another's thoughts, or life-threatening angina. Maybe this is why religious believers have trouble tolerating non-believers in their midst. I've always been surprised at the number of very promising, well-done medical studies that cannot be subsequently confirmed. Independent confirmation has always been considered a scientific gold standard. Perhaps the attitudes and expectations of the researchers should be included in publications, the way funding sources and affiliations are.

It is of course possible that researchers design their studies and evaluate their outcomes to accord with their beliefs. I mean subconsciously, not fraudulently. Still, the research designs and methods are clearly listed in medical papers. It's just that two people using them can come up with different results. Why this happens is an area worthy of study. It affects the drugs and therapies we use every day.

Also worthy of study, *I believe,* are the mechanisms behind the experiences of the people described in this book. If we don't understand things, that doesn't mean they didn't happen. Ignoring or concealing facts is not a scientific accomplishment. Given how common paranormal-type experiences are, and the fact that the people who have them are usually psychiatrically normal (near-death experiencers and children who remember past lives, for example, have been studied and found to be quite mentally intact), we needn't stigmatize the people who've had them.

Nor should we stigmatize the people who try to study them. A university researcher who studies the paranormal is, unfortunately, generally sluicing his or her way right out the door. Federal grant money is basically not available for such research (although a small amount is available for alternative medicine studies).

Perhaps there are things that humankind cannot know. What happens to us after we die might qualify. Michael Faraday, the nineteenth-century British physicist who elucidated many of the relationships between magnetism and electricity (and namesake of the insulated cage mentioned in the previous chapter), felt that some of his work was "upon the threshold of what man is permitted to know in this world." Many would argue that the nuclear physics leading to bomb technology teeters on that same threshold.

But we are curious souls, and changes in the laws of physics reflect an evolution in our concept of reality. As pointed out by Columbia physics professor Brian Greene in a recent *New York Times* editorial, Einstein's $E = mc^2$ is easily derived mathematically. I remember being shown the derivation in a college physics class. The genius of that famous equation lies in its restructuring of reality: Einstein's insight that mass and energy were related, with each capable of becoming the other.

The post–twentieth-century universe contains a number of items that are plainly counterintuitive. From relativity comes the concept that the speed of light is a universal absolute: No matter how fast you are going when you observe it, light always travels at the same speed. Time, on the other hand, is relative. "One person's past could theoretically be another's future" was how it was put at the Einstein exhibit at the American Museum of Natural History. Space, meanwhile, is curved. Some of Einstein's predictions waited decades for the technology that would be able to confirm them. Some wait still. When first published, they were merely "theories."

From quantum mechanics, we know that light and subatomic matter exist both as particles and as waves. From what has come to be called chaos theory, we find that the universe, like the weather, is fundamentally unpredictable.

In Isaac Newton's physics, gravity was a universal force that held the solar system together, and a revolutionary idea at the time. Einstein conceived of gravity as something built-in to the fabric of a universe predictably distorted by objects with mass (like planets, stars, and moons). In 1998, anti-gravity became plausible, as observations showed the universe to be moving apart at an increasingly rapid rate. The March 3, 1998, *New York Times* article about this, "Wary Astronomers Ponder an Accelerating Universe," spoke of the "first strong evidence that the universe is permeated by a repulsive force, the opposite of gravity." A later *Times* piece, "The Mystery of Time" (June 28, 2005), referred to antigravity as a mysterious "dark energy."

It seems that some of nature's energies exist in opposing pairs, as if needed for cosmic balance. Electricity was originally known as static electricity. It was also known that if you rubbed a glass rod with silk, you got a different kind of static electricity from when you rubbed a hard rubber rod with fur. The rubber and glass rods attracted each other; two rubber or two glass rods repelled each other. Benjamin Franklin, seeing the bipolar essence of electricity, named the charge on the glass rod "positive" and that on the rubber one "negative." The connotations of good and evil are coincidental.

I don't know if good and evil in human behavior are really forces, but they're often thought of as such, as if selflessness and selfishness are two opposing poles of the human spirit. I don't know if living things are connected by some natural binding principle. I don't know the answers to the many questions posed in this book. But I would like to know the answers. And apparently, so would a lot of other people.

References

Chapter 2

Cannon, W. B. " 'Voodoo' Death." *American Anthropologist*. 1942; 44:169-181 (reprinted *in American Journal of Public Health* 2002; v. 92(10):1593–6).

Caporael, L. R. "Ergotism: The Satan Loosed in Salem?" *Science*. April 2, 1976; 192(4234): 21–6.

Kandel, E. R., J. H. Schwartz, and T. M. Jessell. "The Hypothalamus Controls the Endocrine System," in *Essentials of Neural Science and Behavior*. Norwalk: Appleton & Lange, 1995. p. 602.

Kirkpatrick, R. A. "Witchcraft and Lupus Erythematosis." *Journal of the American Medical Association*. 1981; 245:1937.

Littlewood, R. L., and C. Douyon. "Clinical Findings in Three Cases of Zombification." *Lancet*. 1997; 350:1094–96

Meador, C. K. "Hex Death: Voodoo Magic or Persuasion?" *Southern Medical Journal*. 1992; 85:244–7.

Steinberg, E. M. "Walter B. Cannon and 'Voodoo Death': A Perspective from 60 Years On." *American Journal of Public Health* 2002; v.92(10):1564–6.

(no author listed). "Puffers, Gourmands, and Zombification." *Lancet.* 1984; 1:1220–1 (editorial).

Chapter 3

Blakemore, C. *Mechanisms of the Mind.* Cambridge: Cambridge University Press, 1977. pp. 49–50.

Duane, T. D., and T. Behrendt. "Extrasensory Electoencephalographic Induction Between Identical Twins." *Science.* 1965; 150:367.

Koren, S. A., and M. A. Persinger. "Possible Disruption of Remote Viewing by Complex Weak Magnetic Fields Around the Stimulus Site and the Possibility of Accessing Real Phase Space: A Pilot Study." *Percept Mot Skills.* 2002; 95:989–98.

Long Island Newsday, Oct. 12, 2004, "Dehydration May Have Saved Teen Trapped in Car for Eight Days," accessed at http://www.newsday.com on Oct. 13, 2004.

Moss, T., H. H. Eveloff, and A. F. Chang. "A Laboratory Investigation of Telepathy: The Study of a Psychic." *Behav Neuropsychiatry.* 1974–1975; 6(1–12):71–80.

Persinger, M. A. "Geophysical Variables and Behavior: LXXI. Differential Contribution of Geomagnetic Activity to Paranormal Experiences Concerning Death and Crisis: An Alternative to the ESP Hypothesis." *Percept Mot Skills.* 1993; 76(2):555–62.

Persinger, M. A., S. A. Koren, and E. W. Tsang. "Enhanced Power Within a Specific Band of Theta Activity in One Person While Another Receives Circumcerebral Pulsed Magnetic Fields: A Mechanism for Cognitive Influence at a Distance?" *Percept Mot Skills.* 2003; 97:877–94.

Persinger, M. A., W. G. Roll, S. G. Tiller, *et al.* "Remote Viewing with the Artist Ingo Swann: Neuropsychological Profile,

Electroencephalographic Correlates, MRI and Possible Mechanisms." *Percept Mot Skills.* 2002; 94(Pt. 1): 927–49.

Radin, D. I. "Event-Related Electroencephalographic Correlations Between Isolated Human Subjects." *J Altern Complement Med.* 2004; 10:315–23.

Standish, L. J. "Electroencephalographic Evidence of Correlated Event-Related Signals Between the Brains of Spatially and Sensory Isolated Human Subjects." *J Altern Complement Med.* 2004; 10:307–14.

Washington Post, Nov. 30, 1995, "Psychic Arms Race Had Several Funding Channels," accessed at http://pqasb.pqarchiver.com on Oct. 8, 2004.

Washington Post, Nov. 29, 1995, "Pentagon Has Spent Millions on Tips from Trio of Psychics: CIA Wants to Shut Down Paranormal Study," accessed at http://pqasb.pqarchiver.com on Oct. 8, 2004.

Chapter 4

Astin, J. A., E. Harkness, and E. Ernst. "The Efficacy of Distant Healing: A Systematic Review of Randomized Trials." *Annals of Internal Medicine.* 2000; 132: 903–10.

Blankfield, R. P., C. Sulzmann, L. G. Fradley, *et al.* "Therapeutic Touch in the Treatment of Carpal Tunnel Syndrome." *J Am Board Fam Pract.* 2001; 14: 335–42.

Byrd, R. C. "Positive Therapeutic Effects of Intercessory Prayer in a Coronary Care Unit Population." *South Med J.* 1988; 81: 826–9.

Gardner, J. W., and J. L. Lyon. "Cancer in Utah Mormon Women by Church Activity Level." *Am J Epidemiol.* 1982; 116: 258–65.

Harkness, E. F., N. C. Abbot, and E. Ernst. "A Randomized Trial of Distant Healing for Skin Warts." *Am J Med.* 2000; 108:507–8.

Harris, W. S., M. Gowda, J. W. Kolb, *et al.* "A Randomized Controlled Trial of the Effects of Remote, Intercessory Prayer on

Outcomes in Patients Admitted to the Coronary Care Unit." *Arch Intern Med.* 1999; 159:2273–8.

Matthews, D. A., S. M. Marlowe, and F. S. MacNutt. "Effect of Intercessory Prayer on Patients with Rheumatoid Arthritis." *South Med J.* 2000; 93:1177–86.

Matthews, W. J., *et al.* "The effects of intercessory prayer, positive visualization and expectancy on the well-being of kidney dialysis patients." *Alternative Therapies in Health and Medicine.* 2001; 7:42–52.

Rosa, L., E. Rosa, L. Sarner, and S. Barrett. "A Close Look at Therapeutic Touch." *JAMA.* 1998; 279:1005–10.

Sicher, F., E. Targ, D. Moore, and H. S. Smith. "A Randomized Double-Blind Study of the Effects of Distant Healing in a Population with Advanced AIDS: Report of a Small-Scale Study." *The Western Journal of Medicine.* 1998; 169:356–63.

Yount, G., J. Solfvin, D. Moore, *et al.* "In Vitro Test of External Qi Gong." *BMC Complementary and Alternative Medicine.* 2004; 4:5.

Chapter 5

Azuonye, I. O. "Diagnosis Made by Hallucinatory Voices." *BMJ.* 1997; 315:1685–86.

Buckley, P. "Mystical Experience and Schizophrenia." *Schizophr Bull.* 1981; 7:516–21.

Du Feu, M., and P. J. McKenna. "Prelingually Profoundly Deaf Schizophrenic Patients Who Hear Voices: A Phenomenological Analysis." *Acta Psychiatr Scand.* 1999; 99:453–59.

Filley, C. M., and B. K. Kelinschmidt-DeMasters. "Neurobehavioral Presentations of Brain Neoplasms." *West J Med.* 1995; 163:19–25.

Honig, A., M. A. Romme, B. J. Ensink, *et al.* "Auditory Hallucinations: A Comparison Between Patients and Nonpatients." *J Nerv Ment Dis.* 1998; 186:646–51.

Johns, L. C., D. Hemsley, and E. Kuipers. "A Comparison of

Auditory Hallucinations in a Psychiatric and No Psychiatric Group." *Br J Clin Psychol.* 2002; 41:81–6.

Kaplan, H. I., and B. J. Sadock. *Kaplan & Sadock's Concise Textbook of Clinical Psychiatry,* 7th ed. Philadelphia: Lippincott, Williams & Wilkins, 2000.

Neppe, V. M. "Tape Recording Auditory Hallucinations." *Am J Psychiatry.* 1988; 145:1316.

Ohayon, M. M. "Prevalence of Hallucinations and Their Pathological Associations in the General Population." *Psychiatry Res.* 2000; 97:153–64.

Schielke, E., E. Reuter, O. Hoffman, *et al.* "Musical Hallucinations with Dorsal Pontine Lesions." *Neurology.* 2000; 55:454–55.

Chapter 6

Etsuko, M. "The Interperetation of Fox Possession: Illness As Metaphor." *Culture, Medicine and Psychiatry.* 1991; 15:453–477.

Garlipp, P., T. Godecke-Koch, D. E. Dietrich, and H. Haltenhof. "Lycanthropy: Psychopathological and Psychodynamic Aspects." *Acta Psychiatrica Scandinavia.* 2004; 109:19–22.

Gomez-Alonzo, J. "Rabies: A Possible Explanation for the Vampire Legend." *Neurology.* 1998; 51:856–9.

Green, R. "Gender Identity in Childhood and Later Sexual Orientation: Follow-Up of 78 Males." *American Journal of Psychiatry.* 1985; 142:339-341.

Illis, L. "On Porphyria and the aetiology of Werewolves." *Proceedings of the Royal Society of Medicine.* 1964; 57:23–6.

Keck, P. E., H. G. Pope, J. I. Hudson, *et al.* "Lycanthropy: Alive and Well in the 20th Century." *Psychological Medicine.* 1988; 18:113–120.

Kulick, A. R., H. G. Pope, and P. E. Keck. "Lycanthropy and Self-Identification." *Journal of Nervous and Mental Disease.* 1990; 178:134–7.

Moselhy, H. F. "Lycanthropy: New Evidence of Its Origin." *Psychopathology.* 1999; 32:173–6.

Wilson, K. K. "The Disparate Classification of Gender and Sexual Orientation in American Psychiatry." Accessed at http://www.priory.con/psych/disparat.htm on Mar. 7, 2005.

Chapter 7

Bozzuto, J. C. "Cinematic Neurosis Following 'The Exorcist.' Report of four cases." *J Nerv Ment Dis.* 1975; 161:43–8.

Freed, R. S., and S. A. Freed. "Ghost illness in a north Indian village." *Social Science and Medicine.* 1990; 30:617–23.

Hale, A. S., and N. R. Pinninti. " Exorcism-resistant ghost possession treated with clopenthixol." *British Journal of Psychiatry.* 1994; 165:386–8.

Kaplan, H. I., and B. J. Sadock. *Kaplan & Sadock's Comprehensive Textbook of Psychiatry*, 6th ed. New York: W. H. Freeman, 1995. pp. 1290–93.

Kaplan, H. I., and B. J. Sadock. *Kaplan & Sadock's Concise Textbook of Clinical Psychiatry*, 2nd ed. Philadelphia: Lippincott Williams & Wilkins, 2004. pp. 266–74.

Salmons, P. H., and D. J. Clarke. "Cacodemonomania." *Psychiatry.* 1987; 50:50–4.

Schendel, E., and R. Kourany. "Cacodemonomania and Exorcism in Children." *J Clin Psychiatry.* 1980; 41:19–23.

Chapter 8

Bobrow, R. S. "The Choice to Die." *Psychology Today.* June 1983; pp. 70–2.

Carey, R. J. "Self-Predicted Fatal Myocardial Infarction in Absence of Coronary Artery Disease." *Lancet.* Jan. 19, 1980; p. 159.

Duncan, J. J., J. E. Farr , S. J. Upton, *et al.* "The Effects of Aerobic Exercise on Plasma Catecholamines and Blood Pressure in Patients with Mild Essential Hypertension." *JAMA.* Nov. 8, 1985; 8;254(18):2609–13.

Engel, G. L. "Sudden and Rapid Death During Psychological Stress." *Annals of Internal Medicine.* 1971; 74:771–82.

McDermott, J. "The Man Who Died on Time." *Life.* Jan. 18, 1960.

Milton, G. W. "Self-Willed Death or the Bone-Pointing Syndrome." *Lancet.* June 23, 1973; p. 1435.

Skala, J. A., and K. E. Freedland. "Death Takes a Raincheck." *Psychosomatic Medicine.* 2004; 66:382–6.

Wittstein, I. S., D. R. Theimann, J. A. C. Lima, *et al.* "Neurohumoral Features of Myocardial Stunning Due to Emotional Stress." *New Engl J Med.* 2005; 352:539–48.

Young, D. C., and E. M. Hade. "Holidays, Birthdays and Postponement of Cancer Death." *JAMA.* 2004; 292:3012–16.

Chapter 9

Blacher, R. S. (in reply) *JAMA.* 1980; 244:30.

Blackmore, S. J. "Near-Death Experiences." *J R Soc Med.* 1996; 89:73–6.

Gallup, G., and W. Proctor. *Adventures in Immortality: A Look Beyond the Threshold of Death.* New York: McGraw-Hill, 1982.

Granqvist, P., M. Fredrikson, P. Unge, *et al.* "Sensed Presence and Mystical Experiences Are Predicted by Suggestibility, Not by the Application of Transcranial Weak Complex Magnetic Fields." *Neuroscience Letters.* 2005; 379:1–6.

Greyson, B. "Dissociation in People Who Have Near-Death Experiences: Out of Their Bodies or Out of Their Minds?" *Lancet.* 2000; 355:460–63.

Greyson, B. "Incidence and Correlates of Near-Death Experience in a Cardiac Care Unit." *Gen Hosp Psychiatry.* 2003; 25:269–76.

—"The Near-Death Experience Scale: Construction, Reliability and Validity." *J Nerv Ment Dis.* 1983; 171:369–75.

—"A Typology of Near-Death Experiences." *Am J Psychiatry.* 1985; 142:967–9.

— "Varieties of Near-Death Experience." *Psychiatry.* 1993; 56:390–9.

Long, J. P. http://www.nderf.org/Physician percent20Survey.htm, accessed Apr. 15, 2005.

Moody, R. A. *Life After Life.* Covington, GA: Mockingbird Books, 1975.

Morse, M. "A Near-Death Experience in a 7-Year-Old Child." *Am J Dis Child.* 1983; 137:95961.

Morse, M. "Childhood Near-Death Experiences." *Am J Dis Child.* 1986; 140:111014.

Noyes, R., and Kletti R. (translation of Von St. Gallen Heim's paper). "The Experience of Dying from Falls." *Omega.* 1972; 3:4552.

Owens, J. E., E. W. Cook, and I. Stevenson. "Features of Near-Death Experience in Relation to Whether or Not Patients Were Near Death. *Lancet.* 1990; 336:1175-77.

Parnia, S., D. G. Walter, R. Yeates, *et al.* "A Qualitative and Quantitative Study of the Incidence, Features and 'tiology of Near Death Experiences in Cardiac Arrest Survivors." *Resuscitation.* 2001; 48:149–56.

Persinger, M. A. "Near-Death Experiences: Determining the Neuroanatomical Pathways by Experiential Patterns and Stimulation in Experimental Settings," in L. Bessette (ed.), *Healing: Beyond Suffering or Death.* Chabanel, Quebec: MNH, 1994. pp. 277–86.

Sabom, M. B. "The Near-Death Experience." *JAMA.* 1980; 244:29–30.

Sabom, M. B., and S. Kreutziger. "Near-Death Experiences." *Journal of the Florida Medical Association,* 1977; 64:648–50.

Van Lommel, P., R. van Wees, V. Meyers, *et al.* "Near-Death Experience in Survivors of Cardiac Arrest: A Prospective Study in the Netherlands." *Lancet.* 2001; 358:2039–45.

Chapter 10

Banaclocha, M. A. "Are Neuronal Activity-Associated Magnetic Fields the Physical Base for Memory?" *Medical Hypotheses.* 2002; 59(5):555–9.

Bengesser, G., and S. Sokoloff. "Antisemitism and Jung's Concept of the Collective Unconscious." *American Journal of Psychiatry.* 1992; 149(3):414–5.

Berg, A. "Ancestor Reverence and Mental Health in South Africa." *Transcultural Psychiatry.* 2003; 40(2):194–207.

Blakemore, C. *Mechanics of the Mind.* Cambridge: Cambridge University Press, 1977.

Dunn, J. R., M. Fuller, J. Zoeger, *et al.* "Magnetic Material in the Human Hippocampus." *Brain Res Bull.* 1995; 36:149–53.

Fonseca, V. S., and L. H. Penna. "The Perspective of the Female Archetype in Nursing." *Rev Bras Enferm.* 2000; 53(2):223–32.

Johnson, N. B. "Primordial Image and the Archetypal Design of Art." *Journal of Analytic Psychology.* 1991; 36(3):371–92.

Kiepenheuer, K. "To Die and To Be! Archetypal View of Puberty Crisis." *Schweiz Arch Neurol Neurochir Psychiatr.* 1984; 134(2):203–13.

Kirschvink, J. L., A. Kobayashi-Kirschvink, and B. J. Woodford. "Magnetite Biomineralization in the Human Brain." *Proc Natl Acad Sci USA.* 1992; 89:7683–7.

Michaud, L. Y., and M. A. Persinger. "Geophysical Variables and Behavior: XXV. Alterations in Memory for a Narrative Following Application of Theta Frequency Electromagnetic Fields." *Perceptual and Motor Skills.* 1985; 60(2):416–8.

Penfield, W. *The Mystery of the Mind.* Princeton: Princeton University Press, 1975. pp.79–80.

Penfield, W., and P. Perot. "The Brain's Record of Auditory and Visual Experience: A Final Summary and Discussion." *Brain.* 1963; 86:595–702.

Schultheiss-Grassi, P. P., R. Wessiken, and J. Dobson. "TEM Investigations of Biogenic Magnetite Extracted from the Human Hippocampus." *Biochim Biophys Acta.* 1999; 1426:212–6.

Storr, A. *Jung.* New York: Routledge, 1973.

Chapter 11

Coons, P. M. "Reports of Satanic Ritual Abuse: Further Implications about Pseudomemories." *Perceptual and Motor Skills.* 1994; 78:1376–8.

Kaplan, H. I., and B. J. Sadock. *Kaplan & Sadock's Concise Textbook of Clinical Psychiatry,* 2nd ed. Philadelphia: Lippincott Williams & Wilkins, 2004. pp. 266–74.

Leavitt, F. "Clinical Correlates of Alleged Satanic Abuse and Less Controversial Sexual Molestation. *Child Abuse and Neglect.* 1994; 18:387–92.

Leavitt, F., and S. M. Labott. "Revision of the Word Association Test for Assessing Associations of Patients Reporting Satanic Ritual Abuse in Childhood." *Journal of Clinical Psychology.* 1998; 54:933–43.

Mazzoni, G. A. L., and E. F. Loftus. "When Dreams Become Reality." *Consciousness and Cognition.* 1996; 5:442–462.

The Milgram Experiment, accessed at http://www.new-life.net/milgram.htm on May 5, 2005.

Ofshe, R. J. "Inadvertent Hypnosis During Interrogation: False Confession Due to Dissociative State; Mis-Identified Multiple Personality and the Satanic Cult Hypothesis." *International Journal of Clinical and Experimental Hypnosis.* 1992; 40:125–56.

Piper, A., and H. Mersky. "The Persistence of Folly: A Critical Examination of Dissociative Identity Disorder. Part I. The Excesses of an Improbable Concept." *Can J Psychiatry.* 2004; 49:592–600.

—"The Persistence of Folly: A Critical Examination of Dissociative Identity Disorder. Part II. The Defence and Decline of Multiple Personality or Dissociative Identity Disorder." *Can J Psychiatry.* 2004; 49:678–83.

Pope, H. G., P. S. Oliva, J. I. Hudson, *et al.* "Attitudes Towards DSM-IV Dissociative Disorders Diagnoses Among Board Certified American Psychiatrists. *Am J Psychiatry.* 1999; 156:321–3.

Putnam, F. C. "The Satanic Ritual Abuse Controversy." *Child Abuse and Neglect.* 1991; 15:175–79.

Sjoberg, R. L. "False Allegations of Sexual Abuse: Case Studies from the Witch Panic in Rattvik 1670–71." *Eur Child Adolesc Psychiatry.* 1997; 6:219–26.

Spanos, N. P., C. A. Burgess, and M. F. Burgess. "Past-Life Identities, UFO Abductions, and Satanic Ritual Abuse: The Social Construction of Memories." *International Journal of Clinical and Experimental Hypnosis.* 1994; XLII:433–46.

Wright, L. "Remembering Satan." *the New Yorker.* May 17, 1993 (pp.60–81) and May 24, 1993 (pp. 54–76).

Young, W. C., R. G. Sachs, B. G. Braun, and R. T. Watkins. "Patients Reporting Ritual Abuse in Childhood: A Clinical Syndrome Report of 37 Cases." *Child Abuse and Neglect.* 1991; 15:181–89.

Chapter 12

Aserinsky, E., and N. Kleitman. "Regularly Occurring Periods of Eye Motility, and Concomitant Phenomena, During Sleep." *Science.* 1953; 118:273–4.

Douglass, A. B., P. Hays, F. Pazderka, *et al.* "Florid Refractory Schizophrenias that Turn Out to Be Treatable Variants of HLA-Associated Narcolepsy." *Journal of Nervous and Mental Disease.* 1991; 179:12–17.

Eiser, A. S. "Physiology and Psychology of Dreams." *Seminars in Neurology.* 2005; 25:97–105.

Goode, E. "Why Do We Sleep?" *New York Times.* Nov. 11, 2003.

Roffwarg, H. P., W. C. Dement, J. N. Muzio, *et al.* "Dream Imagery: Relationship to Rapid Eye Movements of Sleep." *Archives of General Psychiatry.* 1962; 7:235–58.

Shainberg, D. "Telepathy in Psychoanalysis: An Instance." *American Journal of Psychotherapy.* 1976; 30:463–72.

Solms, M. "Dreaming and REM Sleep Are Controlled by Different Brain Mechanisms." *Behavioral and Brain Sciences.* 2000; 23:843–50.

Solms, M. "Meeting comments," accessed at http://web.uct.ac.za/org/rssa/meetings/min03jun.htm on June 3, 2005.

Wolman, B. B., ed. *Handbook of Dreams*. New York: Van Nostrand Reinhold, 1979. pp. 24–5 (the sleep cycle); pp. 168–9 (historical background); pp. 10–11 (the Freudian stream); p. 28, pp. 397–401 (dreams; hallucinations; neurophysiological correlates).

Chapter 13

Gidro-Frank, L, and M. K. Bowersbuch. "A Study of the Plantar Response in Hypnotic Age Regression. *J Nerv Ment Dis*. 1948; 107:443–58.

Gonsalkorale, W. M., V. Miller, *et al.* "Long Term Benefits of Hypnotherapy for Irritable Bowel Syndrome." *Gut*. 2003; 52:1623–9.

LeCron, L. M. "A Study of Age Regression Under Hypnosis," in LeCron, L. M., ed., *Experimental Hypnosis: A Symposium of Articles on Research by Many of the World's Leading Authorities*. New York: Macmillan, 1952. pp. 155–174.

Moss, T., M. J. Paulson, *et al.* "Hypnosis and ESP: A Controlled Experiment." *Am J Clin Hypnosis*. 1970; 13:46–56.

Palsson, O. S., M. J. Turner, D. A. Johnson, *et al.* "Hypnosis Treatment for Severe Irritable Bowel Syndrome: Investigation of Mechanism and Effects on Symptoms." *Dig Dis Sci*. 2002; 11:2605–14.

Radtke, H. L., and N. P. Spanos. "Was I Hypnotized?: A Social Psychological Analysis of Hypnotic Depth Reports." *Psychiatry*. 1981; 44:359–76.

Rausch, V. "Cholecystectomy with Self-Hypnosis." *Am J Clin Hypnosis*. 1980; 22:124–9.

Riskin, J. D., and F. H. Frankel. "A History of Medical Hypnosis." *Psychiatric Clinics of North America*. 1994; 17:601–9.

Sadock, B. J., and V. A. Sadock. *Synopsis of Psychiatry*, 9th ed. Philadelphia: Lippincott Williams & Wilkins, 2003. pp. 960–4.

Stewart, J. H. "Hypnosis in Contemporary Medicine." *Mayo Clin Proc.* 2005; 80:511–24.

Swarbrick, E. T., J. E. Hegarty, L. Bat, *et al.* "Site of Pain from the Irritable Bowel." *Lancet.* 1980; 2:443–6.

Szechtman, H., E. Woody, *et al.* "Where the Imaginal Appears Real: A Positron Emission Tomography Study of Auditory Hallucinations." *Proceedings of the National Academy of Sciences of the USA.* 1998; 95:1956–60.

Vickers, A., and C. Zollman. "Hypnosis and Relaxation Therapies." *BMJ,* 1999; 319:1346–9.

Weitzenhoffer, A. M. *The Practice of Hypnotism,* 2nd ed. New York: John Wiley & Sons, 2000. pp. 3, 245.

Whorwell, P. J., A. Prior, and S. M. Colgan. "Hypnotherapy in Severe Irritable-Bowel Syndrome: Further Experience." *Gut.* 1987; 4:423–5.

Whorwell, P. J., A. Prior, and E. B. Faragher. "Controlled Trial of Hypnotherapy in the Treatment of Severe Refractory Irritable-Bowel Syndrome." *Lancet.* 1984; 2:1232–4.

Wolberg, L. R. *Medical Hypnosis.* New York: Grune & Stratton, 1948. p. 43 (age regression); pp.1–11 (history).

Yapko, M. *Trancework: An Introduction to the Practice of Clinical Hypnosis,* 2nd ed. New York: Brunner/Mazel, 1990.

Chapter 14

Stevenson, I. "A Case of Secondary Personality with Xenoglossy." *Am J Psychiatry.* 1979; 136:1591–2.

Stevenson, I. "A Preliminary Report of a New Case of Responsive Xenoglossy: The case of Gretchen." *Journal of the American Society for Psychical Research.* 1976; 70:65–77.

Stevenson, I. " Xenoglossy; a review and report of a case." *Proceedings of the American Society for Psychical Research.* 1974; 31:1–268.

Stevenson, I. *Unlearned Language: New Studies in Xenoglossy.* Charlottesville: University Press of Virginia, 1984, p. 65.

Zilbergeld, B. *Hypnosis: Questions and Answers.* New York: W. W. Norton, 1986. Chapter 10.

Chapter 15

Hajdu, D. *Positively 4th Street.* New York: Farrar, Strauss and Giroux, 2001. p. 125.

Haraldsson, E. "Personality and Abilities of Children Claiming Previous-Life Memories." *Journal of Nervous and Mental Disease.* 1995; 183:445–51.

King, L. S. "Cases of the Reincarnation Type, Vol. 1: Ten Cases in India" (book review). *JAMA.* 1975; 234:978.

Kolbert, E. "The People's Preacher." *The New Yorker.* Feb. 15 and Feb. 22, 2002.

Stevenson, I. "American Children Who Claim to Remember Previous Lives." *Journal of Nervous and Mental Disease.* 1983; 171:742–8.

—*Children Who Remember Previous Lives*, revised ed. Jefferson, North Carolina: McFarland, 2001.

Chapter 16

Aydin, S., M. Ercan, T. Caskurlu, *et al.* "Acupuncture and Hypnotic Suggestion in the Treatment of Non-Organic Male Sexual Dysfunction." *Scand J Urol Nephrol.* 1997; 31:271–4.

Berman, B. M., L. Lao, P. Langenberg, *et al.* "Effectiveness of Acupuncture as Adjunctive Therapy in Osteoarthritis of the Knee: A Randomized, Controlled Trial." *Ann Intern Med.* 2004; 141:901–10.

Cardini, F., and H. Weixin. "Moxibustion for Correction of Breech Presentation." *JAMA.* 1998; 280:1580–4.

Fireman, Z., A. Segal, Y. Kopelman, *et al.* "Acupuncture Treatment for Irritable Bowel Syndrome: A Double-Blind Controlled Study." *Digestion.* 2001; 64:100–3.

Han, J. S. "Acupuncture and Endorphins." *Neuroscience Letters.* 2004; 361:258–61.

Jeffress, J. E. "Acupuncture: Witchcraft or Wizardry?" *Journal of the American Medical Women's Association.* 1972; 27:519–21.

Kidson, R. *Acupuncture for Everyone.* Rochester, Vermont: Healing Arts Press, 1987. pp. 7–9.

Linde, K., A. Streng, S. Jurgens, *et al.* "Acupuncture for Patients with Migraine." *JAMA.* 2005; 293:2118–25.

Lu, D. P., G. P. Lu, and L. Kleinman. "Acupuncture and Clinical Hypnosis for Facial and Head and Neck Pain: A Single Crossover Comparison." *Am J Clin Hypn.* 2001; 44:141–8.

Manheimer, E., A. White, B. Berman, *et al.* "Meta-Analysis: Acupuncture for Low Back Pain." *Ann Intern Med.* 2005; 142:651–63.

Mann, F. *Acupuncture: The Ancient Art of Chinese Healing and How it Works Scientifically,* 2nd ed. New York: Vintage Books, 1971. pp. 1–2.

Mehl, L. E. "Hypnosis and Conversion of the Breech to the Vertex Presentation." *Arch Fam Med.* 1994; 3:881–7.

Moret, V., A. Forster, M. C. Laverriere, *et al.* "Mechanism of Analgesia Induced by Hypnosis and Acupuncture: Is There a Difference?" *Pain.* 1991; 45:135–40.

NIH Consensus Conference. "Acupuncture." *JAMA.* 1998; 280:1518–24.

Omura, Y. "Impression on Observing Psychic Surgery and Healing in Brazil which Appear to Incorporate (+) Qi Gong Energy & the Use of Acupuncture Points." *Acupunct Electrother Res.* 1997; 22:17–33;

Reichmanis, M., A. Marino, and R. O. Becker. "Electrical Correlates of Acupuncture Points." *IEEE Transactions on Biomedical Engineering.* 1975; 22:533–5.

Research Group of Acupuncture Anesthesia, Peking Medical College. "The Role of Some Neurotransmitters of Brain in Acupuncture Analgesia." *Sci Sin.* 1974; 112–130.

Reston, J. "Now, Let Me Tell You About My Appendectomy in Peking.
. . ." *New York Times*. July 26, 1971, accessed at http://www.acupunc-
ture.com/testimonials/restonexp.htm on Aug. 15, 2005.

Rosen, S. *The Autobiography of Dr. Samuel Rosen*. New York: Alfred A.
Knopf, 1973. pp. 244–6.

Shen, J., N. Wenger, J. Glaspy, *et al.* "Electroacupuncture for
Control of Myeloablative Chemotherapy-Induced Emesis." *JAMA*.
2000; 284:2755–61.

Simmons, M. S., and T. D. Oleson. "Auricular Electrical Stimulation
and Dental Pain Threshold." *Anesth Prog*. 1993; 40:14–9.

Ulett, G. A. "Acupuncture Becomes Scientific." *Skeptical Inquirer*.
March 2003, accessed at http://www.csicop.org/si/2003-
03/acupuncture.html on Aug. 15, 2005.

Vickers, A. J., R. W. Rees, C. E. Zollman, *et al.* "Acupuncture for
Chronic Headache in Primary Care: Large, Pragmatic,
Randomized Trial." *BMJ*. 2004; 328:744.

Chapter 17

Bekenstein, J. B. "Information in the Holographic Universe."
Scientific American. August 2003; 58–65.

Outwater, C., and V. Hamersveld. *Practical Holography*, accessed at
http://www.holo.com/holo//book/book.html on March 30, 2005.

Pribram, K. H. *Languages of the Brain*. Englewood Cliffs: Prentice-
Hall, 1971. pp. 140–166.

Ray, A. L. "Pain Perception in the Older Patient: Using the Pain
Hologram to Understand Neck and Shoulder Pain." *Geriatrics*.
2002; 57:22–6.

Sno, H. N., and D. H. Linszen. "The Déjà Vu Experience:
Remembrance of Things Past?" *American Journal of Psychiatry*.
1990; 147:1587–95.

Chapter 18

Becker, R. O. "The Bioelectric Field Pattern in the Salamander and Its Simulation by an Electric Analog." *IRE Transactions on Medical Electronics.* 1960; ME-7:202–7.

Becker, R. O. *Cross Currents.* Los Angeles: Jeremy P. Tarcher, 1990.

Becker, R. O. "Induced Dedifferentiation: A Possible Alternative to Embryonic Stem Cell Transplants." *NeuroRehabilitation.* 2002; 17:23–31.

Becker, R. O., S. Chapin, and R. Sherry. "Regeneration of the Ventricular Myocardium in Amphibians." *Nature.* 1974; 248:145–7.

Becker, R. O., and G. Selden. *The Body Electric.* New York: Quill (William Morrow), 1985.

Fricker, R. A., M. K. Carpenter, C. Winkler, *et al.* "Site-Specific Migration and Neuronal Differentiation of Human Neural Progenitor Cells after Transplantation in the Adult Rat Brain." *Journal of Neuroscience.* 1999; 19:5990–6005.

Friedman, H., R. O. Becker, and C. H. Bachman. "Direct Current Potentials in Hypnoanalgesia." *Archives of General Psychiatry.* 1962; 7:193–7.

Friedman, H., R. O. Becker, and C. H. Bachman. "Geomagnetic Parameters and Psychiatric Hospital Admissions." *Nature.* 1963; 20:626–8.

Packard, D. S., R. Z. Zheng, and D. C. Turner. "Somite Pattern Regulation in the Avian Segmental Plate Mesoderm. *Development.* 1993; 117:779–791.

Sheldrake, R. *The Sense of Being Stared At.* New York: Crown, 2003. pp. 275–85.

Tian, G. F., H. Azmi, T. Takano, *et al.* "An Astrocytic Basis of Epilepsy." *Nature Medicine.* 2005; 11:973–81.

Zhou, Y., and M. Karplus. "Interpreting the Folding Kinetics of Helical Proteins." *Nature.* 1999; 401:400–3.

Chapter 19

BBC Two. "God on the Brain" program summary. April 17, 2003. Accessed at http://www.bbc.co.uk/science/horizon/2003/godon-brain. shtml on Sept. 30, 2005.

Booth, J. N., S. A. Koren, and M. A. Persinger. "Increased Feelings of the Sensed Presence and Increased Geomagnetic Activity at the Time of the Experience During Exposures to Weak Complex Magnetic Fields." *Int J Neurosci.* 2005; 115:1053–79.

Britton, W. B., and R. R. Bootzin. "Near-Death Experiences and the Temporal Lobe." *Psychol Sci.* 2004; 15:254–8.

Cook, C. M., and M. A. Persinger. "Experimental Induction of the 'Sensed Presence' in Normal Subjects and an Exceptional Subject." *Percept Mot Skills.* 1997; 85:683–93.

Derr, J. S., and M. A. Persinger. "Geophysical Variables and Behavior: LIV. Zeitoun (Egypt) Apparitions of the Virgin Mary as Tectonic Strain-Induced Luminosities." *Percept Mot Skills.* 1989; 68:123–8.

Fournier, N. M., and M. A. Persinger. "Geophysical Variables and Behavior: C. Increased Geomagnetic Activity on Days of Commercial Air Crashes Attributed to Computer or Pilot Error but Not Mechanical Failure." *Percept Mot Skills.* 2004; 3 (pt. 2):19–24.

Gearhart, L., and M. A. Persinger. "Geophysical Variables and Behavior. XXXIII. Onsets of Historical and Contemporary Poltergeist Episodes Occurred with Sudden Increases in Geomagnetic Activity." *Percept Mot Skills.* 1986; 62:463–6.

Granqvist, P., M. Fredrikson, P. Unge, *et al.* "Sensed Presence and Mystical Experiences Are Predicted by Suggestibility, Not by Application of Transcranial Weak Complex Magnetic Fields." *Neuroscience Letters.* 2005; 379:1–6.

Grandqvist, P., *et al.* "Reply to M. A. Persinger and S. A. Koren's response to Grandqvist *et al.*" *Neuroscience Letters.* 2005; 380:348–50.

Healey, F., and M. A. Persinger. "Experimental Production of Illusory (False) Memories in Reconstructions of Narratives: Effect

Size and Potential Mediation by Right Hemispheric Stimulation from Complex, Weak Magnetic Fields." *Int J Neurosci.* 2001; 106:195–207.

Hercz, R. "The God Helmet." *Saturday Night* magazine, pp. 40–6. Accessed at http://www.geocities.com/satanicus_2/GodHelmet.html? 200530 on Sept. 30, 2005.

Hitt, J. "This is Your Brain on God." *Wired.* Nov. 1999; issue 7.11. Accessed at http://www.wired.com/wired/archive/7.11/persinger_pr.html on Sept. 30, 2005.

Jaynes, J. *The Origin of Consciousness in the Breakdown of the Bicameral Mind.* Boston: Houghton Mifflin, 1977.

Mesulam, M. M. "Dissociative States with Abnormal Temporal Lobe EEG." *Arch Neurol.* 1981; 38:176–181.

Morneau, D. M., D. A. MacDonald, and C. J. Holland. "A Confirmatory Study of the Relation Between Self-Reported Complex Partial Epileptic Signs, Peak Experiences and Paranormal Beliefs." *Br J Clin Psychol.* 1996; 35:627–30.

The Natural Connection. *The UFO Machine.* Accessed at http://www.natural-connection.com/resource/spectrum.html on Sept. 30, 2005.

O'Connor, R. P., and M. A. Persinger. "Geophysical Variables and Behavior: LXXXII. A Strong Association Between Sudden Infant Death Syndrome and Increments of Global Geomagnetic Activity—Possible Support for the Melatonin Hypothesis. *Percept Mot Skills.* 1997; 84:395–402.

Persinger, M. A. "Feelings of Past Lives as Expected Perturbations Within the Neurocognitive Processes that Generate the Sense of Self: Contributions from Limbic Lability and Vectorial Hemisphericity." *Percept Mot Skills.* 1996; 83:1107–21.

—"The Neuropsychiatry of Paranormal Experiences." *J Neuropsychiatry Clin Neurosci.* 2001; 13:515–35.

Persinger, M. A., and J. S. Derr. "Geophysical Variables and Behavior: XXIII. Relations Between UFO Reports Within the

Uinta Basin and Local Seismicity." *Percept Mot Skills*. 1985; 60:143–52.

Persinger, M. A., and S. A. Koren. "Experiences of Spiritual Visitation and Impregnation: Potential Induction by Frequency-Modulated Transients from an Adjacent Clock." *Percept Mot Skills*. 2001; 92:35–6.

— "A Response to Grandqvist *et al.*" (letter). *Neuroscience Letters*. 2005; 380:346–7.

Persinger, M. A., S. A. Koren, and R. P. O'Connor. "Geophysical Variables and Behavior: CIV. Power-Frequency Magnetic Field Transients (5 Microtesla) and Reports of Haunt Experiences Within an Electronically Dense House." *Percept Mot Skills*. 2001; 92:673–4.

Persinger, M. A., and R. P. O'Connor. "Geophysical Variables and Behavior. CIII. Days with Sudden Infant Deaths and Cardiac Arrhythmias in Adults Share a Factor with PC1 Geomagnetic Pulsations: Implications for Pursuing Mechanism." *Percept Mot Skills*. 2001; 92:653–4.

Persinger, M. A., S. G. Tiller, and S. A. Koren. "Experimental Simulation of a Haunt Experience and Elicitation of Paroxysmal Electroencephalographic Activity by Transcerebral Complex Magnetic Fields: Induction of a Synthetic 'Ghost'?" *Percept Mot Skills*. 2000; 90:659–74.

Persinger, M. A., and P. M. Valliant. "Temporal Lobe Signs and Reports of Subjective Paranormal Experiences in a Normal Population: A Replication." *Percept Mot Skills*. 1985; 60: 903–9.

Sadler, R. M., and S. Rahey. "Prescience as an Aura of Temporal Lobe Epilepsy." *Epilepsia*. 2004; 45:982–4.

Suess, L. A., and M. A. Persinger. "Geophysical Variables and Behavior: XCVI. 'Experiences' Attributed to Christ and Mary at Marmora, Ontario, Canada May Have Been Consequences of Environmental Electromagnetic Stimulation: Implications for Religious Movements." *Percept Mot Skills*. 2001; 93:435–50.

Zeman, A. "Tales from the Temporal Lobes." *N Engl J Med.* 2005; 352:119–21.

Chapter 20

Benson, H., and D. P. McCallie, Jr. "Angina Pectoris and the Placebo Effect." *New England Journal of Medicine.* 1979; 300:1424–8.

Carrel, A. *The Voyage to Lourdes.* New York: Harper & Bros., 1950.

Dean, S. R., C. O. Plyler, Jr., and M. L. Dean. "Should Psychic Studies Be Included in Psychiatric Education? An Opinion Survey." *Psychiatry.* 1980; 137:1247–9.

Eisenberg, D. M., R. C. Kessler, C. Foster, *et al.* "Unconventional Medicine in the United States: Prevalence, Costs, and Patterns of Use." *New England Journal of Medicine.* 1993; 328:246–52.

Faraday quote in: Roach, M. *Spook.* New York: W.W. Norton, 2005. p. 202.

Greene, B. "That Famous Equation and You." *New York Times.* Sept. 30, 2005.

Horrigan, B. "Marilyn Schlitz, Ph.D., on Consciousness, Causation and Evolution" (interview). *Alternative Therapies.* 1998; 4:82–90.

Overbye, D. "Remembrance of Things Future: The Mystery of Time." *New York Times.* June 28, 2005.

Wilford, J. N. "Wary Astronomers Ponder an Accelerating Universe." *New York Times.* March 3, 1998.

Index